Obesity Kills

Fight It and Survive It

Jason Woodward

Table of Contents

Introduction

Our world is fighting malnutrition and obesity at the same time. It's very common to express concern for those who are dying of hunger, as one should. However, people seem to forget the dreaded disease of obesity because it's not an instant and painful death. Obesity is a problem of excessive choice while hunger and malnutrition are a lack of choice. As we raise awareness to end world hunger, it's also important to highlight the causes, effects, and struggles of obesity spreading around the world.

In fact, our world is seeing more deaths from obesity than from malnutrition in most parts of the world. Obesity has even started in parts of Africa, where 24% of the children—under 5—are obese (World Health Organization, 2021). These numbers are becoming increasingly alarming to every individual. The World Obesity Atlas (2022) predicts that by 2030, 1 billion people will be obese globally. We cannot just sit by and watch as the world suffers from excessiveness while some people out there die from malnutrition. Unlike many other problems in the world, obesity is in our hands. We can all act—by helping ourselves, someone we care about, or by simply being aware. Obesity can be cured with the right knowledge and dedication.

While obesity comes from overeating and not exercising, there are many more reasons people gain weight in today's world. Reasons can vary from family issues, mental health issues, and even the world's problems. For example, Covid-19 took a toll on all our mental health. And many stress factors can lead to an unhealthy lifestyle that in turn increases obesity. Consequently, during the pandemic people with obesity were at a higher risk. According to the Centers of Disease Control and

Prevention (CDC), the chances of obese people getting admitted to hospitals due to Covid-19 is three times more than healthy people (2020).

Other than the pandemic, obesity can be inherited from genetics and can also depend on environmental and psychological factors. That will all be covered in detail further in this book.

It's important to remember that obesity is not to be taken lightly because it's killing you slowly, and even though you might not feel it now, you will very soon if you don't act. The most probable impact obesity has is heart attacks and heart failure. But with obesity, you have the upper hand. You're in control of your mind and body; if you dedicate yourself to getting out of obesity, then you can. You're not stuck in this forever. All it requires from you is dedication and hard work to get healthier and live a happy life.

Don't forget to seek help whenever needed. When we suffer from any medical issue, we see the doctor and that applies here as well. It's always advised to seek medical help, so you can detect the cause of obesity, and how you can move forward. For example, obesity caused by genetics will have to be treated differently compared to obesity from excessive eating or obesity from issues affecting our mental capacity. Each approach will be unique in every way, and while we are going to cover them all in this book, it's important that you're diagnosed correctly, so you can know where to start, and what to do.

To give some boost, let's hear from some people, who are dealing or have dealt with obesity, to get a better perspective. Taken from The World Obesity Atlas (2022):

Ogweno Stephen, CEO of Stowelink Inc. in Kenya said:

> I was born with childhood obesity, and if statistics are anything to go by, by the time I was 18, I was supposed to be living with full-blown obesity. By the time I was 25, I was supposed to have developed hypertension, and by the time I was 35, I probably would have developed diabetes resulting from obesity. But this was not the case because early in my life I had people close to me who understood that obesity was a disease and helped me

manage my condition. Now I realize that this is a privilege that not a lot of people—especially in sub-Saharan Africa—have when it comes to obesity. I developed an organization called Stowelink, and from 2016, we have been educating communities about obesity. This is grassroots-level action, but action on obesity is multifaceted, and it needs everybody. (p. 8)

Allison Ibrahim from Kuwait shared her experience:

I gained a considerable amount of weight with my first pregnancy (my son is now 31). Since then, I have lost 60 lbs., and I'm very proud of the hard work that I put in to do that. But it doesn't stay that way without supportive systems in place; without healthcare professionals who understand the needs of a person living with obesity and other chronic conditions. If you have a medical team that works with you, and if you're an advocate for yourself and have education available, you can try to live a somewhat healthy lifestyle. Without help from the global community, it's a challenge. We need everyone's help, and everyone's understanding. Weight stigma, weight bias, is not acceptable. (p. 8)

These stories are just the beginning and show us that people have come out of obesity from different situations, and if they can, you can too. Prioritizing your health is vital, and once you use that as your motivation, you will be able to move mountains.

People all over the world have fought obesity and are still doing so; ultimately, they can live a much healthier and happier life. This book will help you get inside the information on how to get out of obesity, so you can put an end to it for yourself or your loved ones. Having awareness of the causes and impacts can also do a lot of good to the people around you. You might ask these questions yourself. How do I know if I/they are obese? How did I/they gain weight and become obese? What are the risks of being obese? How can I help myself or someone I love?

Obesity Kills targets obese people of different age groups, their families, and their friends. The goal of the book is for the readers to receive:

- The reasons behind being obese.
- Vision that obesity is unhealthy.
- Knowledge about a healthy diet with portion control to shed weight.
- Insight into the health issues caused by obesity.
- Awareness of the health problems that are avertable.
- Ways to manage the inevitable health problems associated with obesity.
- Tips to maintain good health.
- Interest in self-care and personal health.
- Realization that obesity reduces life expectancy.
- Warning about the risks of heart attack and stroke due to obesity.
- Understanding the importance of socializing to maintain sound mental health.
- Ability to recognize a health emergency, and the right time to seek medical aid.
- Motivation to work toward addressing any issues that lead to obesity.
- Information that obesity is far more expensive.

Chapter 1:
Don't Ignore Childhood Obesity

The rise of childhood obesity has placed the health of an entire generation at risk. –
Tom Vilsack

Living a lavish life can sometimes be the reason for being overweight or obese. Statistically, 12.7 million children in the United States are obese (American Academy of Child and Adolescent Psychiatry, 2016). Living in a first-world country and growing up in a pampered household may sound like a dream for most, but it comes with its own problems. The most common reasons for obesity in children are the lack of exercise and the availability of whatever they want. This may sound harsh, but when you give your children everything they want, whether it's eating out every day or buying them gadgets that keep them at home, you're subconsciously encouraging them to be lazy, increasing their chances of becoming obese.

Parents, even though they may have the best interest in mind for their kids, sometimes tend to ignore the early signs of obesity that can cause your child serious health problems from early in life. Aside from the drastic health problems that they're going to face, they will also face mental health issues. So, when you see the signs, don't turn a blind eye for the sake of your child; instead identify the reason, become aware of the impacts it will have on your child's mental and physical health, and know the different ways you can help your child fight obesity.

Reasons for Childhood Obesity

The first and most common reason is the lifestyle we live in. The more comfortable with technology we become, the more we rely on others and not ourselves, and the more we start to get lazy and gain weight. Obesity won't come at you and punch you in the face but will slowly creep into your body without you noticing it. It can very easily start with your child gaining some weight, but when it gets out of hand and becomes obesity, you will never know unless you keep track of your child. Sometimes, parents who are working find it hard to keep track of their child and start leaving them alone more often with gadgets. They don't know how unhealthy it gets for the child. The easiest way you can find out if your child is obese or getting there is by noticing their daily lifestyle. What do they eat in a day? What do they do in a day? Are they eating only three meals a day, or is there constant munching throughout the day? Is your child going out to play, going for a walk, or cycling, or are they just staring at screens all day long?

Once you ask yourself these questions, you can get closer to identifying the main reason why your child is gaining weight, and what help you need to seek for your child to become healthier.

In today's world, it's getting extremely easy to consume what you want, and it's affordable. But what kinds of food are the most affordable? As an average person, the increasing amounts of fast-food advertising can seem like an affordable way to eat, but those foods are the ones that can make your child obese. It may be delicious and addictive, but the unhealthy factor can cost you your life. A child who is school-going should have an average calorie intake of 1,500–2,500. A McDonald's cheeseburger meal alone is 800 calories and above. Considering that your child frequently consumes fast foods at least 5 times a week, that will make their daily calorie count exceed the average limit, and they will start gaining weight. So, a cheap meal is going to cost you your child's physical health.

Moreover, a lack of exercise can also lead your child down the road of obesity. As mentioned briefly above, we have all become dependent on technology today. But it was not always like this. When we were in our childhood years, we used to go out with our friends, cycle to school, or even just be out in our backyards jumping about. However, children now don't go out to play; they play on their laptops and other screens. They don't jump about in the playground; they play games where the character does the jumping for them. This causes them to miss out on exercise, and the fat in their bodies to accumulate to the point where they become obese.

Another reason why your child might have obesity could be due to family history. If obesity and being overweight run in your family, you should be extra careful with your child because they may inherit the genes and easily form habits that can make them obese.

Medical Issues From Obesity

Your child, if diagnosed with obesity, will likely face most of these medical impacts listed below:

Type-2 Diabetes

Type-2 diabetes can be inherited from the family and can also be a result of obesity. This type of diabetes is a condition when your body cannot metabolize glucose and might need help from medicines and injections to get the glucose metabolized. Eating too much sugar can then become a death sentence as you may face several more issues. According to DiabetesTalk, you increase your chances of blindness, amputation, kidney failure, heart attack, stroke, gum disease, and high blood pressure (Staff, 2018). However, if you're diagnosed with diabetes, there's no cure, and you must be cautious of your lifestyle choices for the rest of your life. That's why it's a real danger to your kid, especially if they're obese, to get diagnosed with type-2 diabetes.

High Cholesterol and Blood Pressure

It's a given that when your child gets diagnosed with obesity, they will face cholesterol or blood pressure issues in the future. High cholesterol develops fats in the form of deposits in your blood vessels, restricting the blood flow to your child's body parts that can cause them a lot of problems—health wise. Your child will feel immense pain in their chest and can be introduced to heart problems and increase the possibility of getting a heart attack. Moreover, they can also suffer from a stroke when their cholesterol levels are high as the blood flow to the brain suffers or gets blocked.

High blood pressure can also be an effect of obesity. This happens when the blood flowing through your veins is constantly at a high pressure or force. What high blood pressure does is weaken your arteries and muscles, weakening your heart. Again, leading to heart failure or attacks accompanied by kidney failure. High blood pressure also lowers the chances of performing sexually and can cause your child problems in the future.

These two are the most common impacts of obesity and should be taken very seriously. You can indeed reverse the effects with medical help and being in good shape that also means fighting obesity, that's the root of all these problems.

Asthma or Breathing Problems

Another impact of obesity is that some find it difficult to breathe. And not like after running three laps, but you can also find it hard to breathe after climbing a flight of stairs or after a short jog, especially if you're obese. Getting asthma is not something that's very common because of obesity, but there have been studies ongoing about this. And while asthma may be more of a genetic complication, obesity can make it worse and can even cause breathing problems that can then lead to asthmatic attacks.

Having breathing problems also makes it harder to exercise and get fit. And the longer you ignore your child's obesity, the more difficult it will be for them to exercise and regain their health. So, when you see the symptoms of obesity, it's important that you make them exercise and get moving, so the breathing problems can be controlled.

Sleep Disorders

A study was conducted with 70 children to test whether obesity affected their sleep patterns. The children were all tested for any other disorders or problems that may have caused them to have sleep disorders and were separated. After random selection, they concluded that being overweight did, in fact, give the children a hard time while sleeping (Bakalar, 2009).

Being an obese child with sleep disorders can really disturb your child's mind and body. Children's sleep is the most important part of their lives, and it's highly stated that children require a minimum of eight hours of sleep. When that sleep time is sacrificed, your child will fall behind, become lethargic, and most probably, develop an attitude change.

This does not just mean having minor sleeping problems; it, in fact, implies that your child could also be diagnosed with sleep apnea. As if obesity is not enough, developing sleep apnea is just going to make it worse for your child. Sleep apnea is a condition where your child will wake up frequently in the night resulting in irregular sleep patterns; they may snore or make noises that may make others think they're choking in their sleep (Suni, 2019). This can cause your child to develop headaches and engage in frequent daytime napping to recover what they lose at night.

Heart Disorders

By ignoring childhood obesity, you're signing your kid up for a lifetime of heart problems. Even if your child gets lucky and doesn't die from the heart attacks that will haunt them for the rest of their life, they will have to endure a lifetime of heart disorders. It might be too late for them to help themselves if you don't help them from the start. We're not just talking about problems later in their lives, but if you fail to help them when you notice obesity symptoms, then you're signing them up for immediate heart problems. Thomas Kimball, Professor of Pediatrics at the University of Cincinnati College of Medicine, confirms that risks associated with childhood obesity are immediate and not down the road in adulthood (Doheny, 2009).

Social Challenges

Aside from the dire consequences of obesity that your child will face, they will also face plenty of social challenges and mental health issues.

Isolation and Loneliness

When your child struggles with obesity and weight issues, they're bound to face difficulties fitting in with people. This might cause them to isolate themselves, either willingly or by force, and find themselves lonely very often. They might even feel like they have no one to talk to openly. Psychologically, once they don't find themselves fitting in with social groups, they may find it very hard to trust people, even later in life. As an immediate effect, they may want to drop out of school and hang out just in their room, where they won't feel left out (Social Isolation, Obesity, and Health, 2013). This can also affect their ability to interact socially with people. Isolation and loneliness can also lead to other illnesses that can target your child. There has been successful research conducted to show the linkage between social isolation and early death and failure (Yang et al., 2013).

Bullying

While there are sensitive people out there with awareness, your child may still face bullying for their weight. They may or may not be able to do anything about it, but it will surely have a negative mental impact on your child. Bullying can make them feel as though they are what their weight is, and that they're not enough. And it can also lead to them losing confidence in themselves, and their self-esteem dropping to its lowest. Once they get bullied, they may find it hard to make friends or trust anyone easily. While this is not entirely their fault, but also yours as a parent; ignoring their health can also cost them in school or when they go out. Mental strain like this can make your child seek unhealthy ways to get slim later in life, making themselves even weaker and can lead to many other issues of desperation.

Depression

Obese children had a 95% higher risk of depression than healthy children in one study (Sutaria et al., 2018). Obesity doesn't just affect the body but also the mind. At a young age, when faced with such complex situations in their lives, regarding physical and mental health, can make your child feel heavy and depressed. It can change their outlook on life to a negative one increasing their thoughts of self-harm or suicide. That's why it's critical that you notice their signs of obesity and work hard alongside them to make their lives healthy and happy again.

How to Help Your Child

As mentioned above, when you have even the slightest concern of obesity in your child, seek medical help and try to help them. Here are some things you, as a parent, can do.

Create Awareness About Childhood Obesity

The first step in helping your child overcome obesity is to be aware of it and acknowledge it. Turning a blind eye or calling your child out as if it's entirely their fault is not going to help them get fit. You must make them accept their condition first before moving onto the consequences. You don't have to scare them; you must motivate them to change and work hard to lead a healthy life. So, before you do anything, sit with your child, and talk them through what they're going to need to do; how they will do it; and how you're going to be there to help and support them unconditionally, so they can live a long and fulfilled life.

Encourage Physical Activities

Get them moving and not right into strenuous workouts, but a simple jog or a bike ride to and from school. You can also take them out for adventurous activities more often to make them enjoy losing weight. Remember that they're still children, and don't need the extra pressure of going to the gym and losing weight on top of their school and social life. Instead, after they finish school, encourage them to participate in activities that are of interest to them and will keep them moving. As previously stated, one of the causes of obesity is that people are constantly eating with no physical activity to burn off that fat; therefore, encourage them to try out for football or basketball where they can have fun while moving around. Moreover, you can make them do household chores that can get them occupied away from being cooped up in their rooms.

There's so much more you, as parents, can do to ensure that your child is not under too much pressure, but is still determined to lose that excess weight and become healthy and fit. If you force them to work out or pressure them too much, they may not be motivated to lose that weight, and instead, go the opposite way of getting healthier, or might take unhealthy routes to get fit that will make their life worse.

Introduce Healthy Eating Habits

Get them to eat healthier and reduce their snacking frequency slowly. This doesn't mean that they must only eat vegetables and fruits all the time; no, you can introduce healthier versions of the foods they love. For example, if they like chips, there are healthy ones made that are not fried in oil. Just because they must lose weight doesn't mean they have to stop having fun. In fact, you can even go out to eat on the weekends. The only important things to remember are to have more healthy foods during meals; limit their snacking frequency; and decrease their eating of unhealthy foods, slowly and gradually. One way you can do this is by creating healthier habits among the family. When they're expected to eat healthy, it's impossible to separate them while eating unhealthy foods yourself. The best way to make them feel comfortable eating healthier foods is by doing it as a family, so they get the mental support and cheering that they require.

Always Be There

As mentioned above, you can show your support in numerous ways. Show them that you care about them and are there to back them up whenever they need it. This also includes emotional cheering. As such, when on this journey to fight obesity, your child will require you to understand how hard it is for them, and you will have to give them the freedom to breathe. If they want to go out to eat their favorite foods with their friends, let them go occasionally. Don't cage them in, making them think it's best for themselves because then that will make it hard for them to socialize in the future. Consequently, it turns them back to obesity again.

Chapter 2:

Why Do People Become Overweight

To be able to identify and fight obesity, you must be able to recognize the exact cause of your weight gain. Sometimes, it's just one factor, and sometimes, it's more than one; nonetheless, you should have proper knowledge of the factors. Let's investigate some of them below.

Lifestyle Choices

In today's world, we have hopped on too many trends, thinking they're cool, and have forgotten our traditions and culture. Some of those choices can also cause obesity.

Eating Habits

There are so many instances that make us turn to fast foods and unhealthy options. Sometimes, it's being too busy to cook healthy food, or that unhealthier options are easy to find or make, or even the availability or lack of money to help decide where and what to eat. Unhealthy options are so easily available and at an affordable price that you may think you're saving up by eating cheap, but consuming those processed, sugary, and high-calorie foods is going to cost you physically, mentally, and even financially in your life.

Then, there's the whole snacking equation that can even throw a healthy person off. It could be the snaking of popcorn drowned in butter or the mid-meeting snack of something equally damaging but tasty. While this is acceptable occasionally, it can cause serious harm to your body otherwise. Obesity, even though dire, could become the least of your worries. We require three proper meals per day and adding snacks to that as a habit could increase your calorie count, therefore, increasing weight and causing obesity. On average, a female adult requires 1,600–2,000 calories per day, and an adult male requires 2,200–3,000 calories per day (Davidson, 2021). Once you exceed those numbers frequently, you will see yourself gaining weight rapidly.

Inactive Regime

As discussed in the previous chapter, when we eat—even the normal amount—but don't exercise and move about, the energy gets stored in the form of fat that makes us gain weight. This can also be the cause of obesity for those who sit in their office and work for most hours, then go home and relax again by sitting and watching TV, and then going to sleep. This cause has escalated the weight gain during the pandemic. According to a study at Harvard Health, there was a 39% weight gain in America, which was above the normal fluctuation of 2.5 pounds (MD, 2021).

Obesity rates increased during the pandemic due to less activity in our daily lives in the form of exercise. We think that eating fewer calories in a day without exercise won't let us gain weight, but the human body is made for movement. We're not meant to be sitting on our butts every day. That's why, even if you have a desk job, you must find a way to become more physically active apart from that. Going for a walk, jog, or run daily may seem like a hassle with slow results, but it benefits you in the long term.

Undisciplined

There can also be instances when you find yourself eating healthy meals regularly, but still find yourself gaining weight. This can be due to skipping meals or munching frequently. If you think that skipping meals will help you lose weight, then you might just find yourself down the opposite road. Because without a diet to follow, if you try to skip meals, you will find yourself hungry more resulting in you munching on snacks with a lot of sugar for energy, and when you approach the next meal, you will overeat. That just might not compensate for the meal you skipped.

Losing weight doesn't mean you skip meals and munch instead. Rather, eat these proper and healthy meals every day to control your weight gain. Eating such meals at the right time will also reduce your hunger and won't have you munching on unhealthy snacks more often. So, discipline is very important when on the journey of controlling your weight.

Health-Related Problems

Sometimes, it's not our choices that make us gain weight. There are certain times when our health problems can also result in weight gain. Such health problems could be due to genetics, or something you have been suffering from for a while.

Binge-Eating Disorder (BED)

Known as the most common disorder in the United States, BED is a problem, and while treatable, can be life-threatening, and is the biggest contributor to obesity. When diagnosed with BED, you might find yourself hungry every two hours, or find yourself losing control when you start to eat—eating in bigger quantities than usual. You may find yourself eating quicker than normal, eating until you can't move, eating a lot even when you're not hungry, and feeling guilty and ashamed after it. There are many reasons someone may turn to binge-eating, and most of them revolve around mental pressure from within or from others. This disorder has a very direct link to obesity that can make your life even worse.

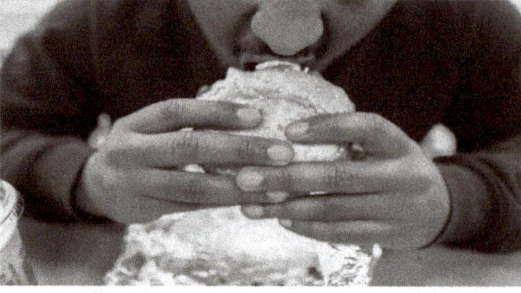

Thyroid Disorder

This disease can be inherited from family members or can also be developed otherwise. A thyroid disorder is when your thyroid—located near your windpipe—either functions more or less than usual. Gaining weight happens when your thyroid doesn't function properly. Since this body part controls how your metabolism works by releasing a thyroid hormone, if that is not released at the right amount, you can suffer from hypothyroidism. This causes the hormone to not release properly, and thus, makes your metabolism low. So, when you eat, not all your food gets converted into energy and can instead cause you to gain weight.

Depression

Depression and obesity are a vicious cycle that can engulf many people. There have been studies that prove obesity is due to depression, and depression is due to obesity (Fuller et al., 2017). When people feel down and feel like there's no more hope left for them in the world, they very often tend to seek comfort in food. When socializing and going out become pointless, people turn to food to make themselves feel better.

Sometimes, that may work, but it also increases the chance of you gaining weight and becoming obese.

Cushing Syndrome

Cushing syndrome is another disease that can cause weight gain. This syndrome occurs when your body starts producing high levels of the hormone cortisol. Cortisol is a vital hormone that handles a lot of roles in your body including the conversion of fats and carbohydrates into energy, responding to stress, regulating blood pressure, and so much more. Not only do the effects of this syndrome include weight gain, but you will also notice fatty deposits on your face; stretch marks starting to form near your stomach and thighs; and your skin becoming prone to bruising.

Insomnia

Studies are being conducted and data is being gathered on how a person's inability to get adequate sleep contributes to obesity (Crönlein, 2016). Hormones in your body start to fluctuate when sleep is not sufficient. The hormones ghrelin and leptin—which control your hunger—start rapidly fluctuating, making you more likely to snack frequently and on unhealthy options; therefore, increasing the chance of obesity for you. It's vital that you take extra precaution, especially if you have insomnia.

Because obesity is an easy train to catch, and that can then introduce you to new sleeping problems and others too.

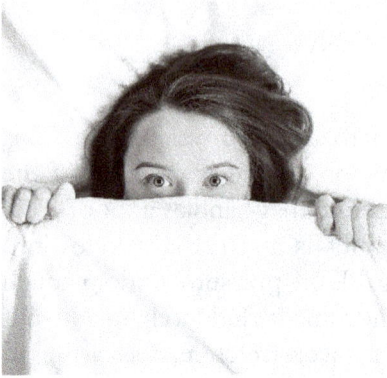

Emotional Imbalance

When we're not healthy mentally, we cannot expect to be physically fit as well. There are times when we're so stressed in life that we either eat too much or too little with no in between. People also seek relief with food when they're stressed by taking multiple breaks and turning to a snack. There are also times when we lose all hope of the situation, turn negative, and indulge in our comfort food to make us feel better. In return, we feel guilty and ashamed of eating until we're uncomfortably full.

Other than stress, we also gain weight when we're not confident in our own bodies and lives. Low self-esteem makes us turn to comfort food whenever there's a slight mishap. When you begin to love yourself, you start to take the best possible care of your physical and mental health; however, the opposite is true when you don't love yourself. You don't find yourself worthy of taking proper care of yourself and might go down the slippery road of gaining weight and becoming obese.

Genetic Disorders

These genetic disorders mentioned below are some of the main ones that will most definitely cause weight gain. Because of the weight gain, other problems follow.

Bardet-Biedl Syndrome

While the most common impact of this syndrome is vision loss, obesity is also an effect of Bardet-Biedl syndrome. These inherited diseases can affect one or many parts of a person's body, that's why it's important to get yourself diagnosed if anyone in your family has this syndrome. Weight gain from this syndrome will also increase your chances of developing diabetes, high cholesterol, and high blood pressure.

Prader-Willi Syndrome

People with this syndrome develop a hunger that's never satisfied. That's why they eat but never feel full. This causes them to gain weight because they have a hard time controlling themselves, and most of the time, don't even know when to stop. It's very important that people diagnosed with this syndrome seek medical help, and those who are unsure should get themselves checked out. Because this syndrome will cause obesity and many other conditions that follow.

Other Factors

Let us look at other factors that may not relate to medical and mental issues but may cause weight gain.

Pregnancy

It's natural for the mother to gain weight from pregnancy to be able to support and keep the baby healthy for the term it's inside her. Since you gain weight during your pregnancy, the weight won't magically go away after birth. But before we dive into that, let's look deeper into weight gain during pregnancy. Pregnant people should keep in touch with their doctors frequently and monitor their weight gain too. And if the weight gained is too little, then the complication during birth could be that the baby will be too small and underdeveloped. However, if the weight gain is too much, then the mother can face complications during birth as the baby will be too big, and she might have to go through a cesarean procedure. Moreover, the baby and the mother could face obesity later.

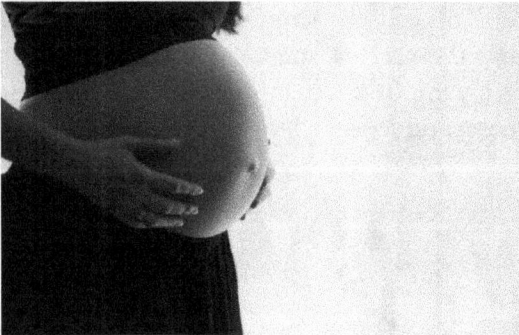

Lack of Awareness

Knowing your body's average body-mass index (BMI), the number of calories you need to consume each day, and the nutritional facts of your foods is critical for preventing weight gain. If such knowledge is lacking, then you might find yourself gaining weight even if you eat lots of healthy food daily and very little junk food. Your BMI can be easily found on the internet with information about your age, gender, weight, and height. If not, you can also seek medical help. Your average calorie count can be figured out similarly. There are numerous apps that will not only help you find your average calorie count but will also calculate your daily count based on what you ate. This can also be done manually by checking the nutritional facts of foods that are already packaged, and by having a general idea of the calories you find in fresh fruits and vegetables.

Chapter   3:
Different Categories of Obesity

Finding out the category of obesity is highly important in treating it and helping someone as well. A researcher at Massachusetts General Hospital told The New York Times that there are 59 categories of obesity (Kaplan, 2016). The most important reason to know which category of obesity is affecting you is so you can find the most effective way to treat it. Not all diagnoses will work for all types of obesity levels. Some may work at one level while some may not.

You may have also tried one way to lose weight but found it very difficult to do so. It's because you might be doing the wrong exercise to lose weight or are doing exercise for the body part where you may have the least fat deposition. Knowing the different categories will also help keep you motivated to lose weight as you will see the right number of results based on the type of obesity you have. There are two ways you can identify which category of obesity you fit into. One is based on the place you notice fat deposition, and one is by calculating your BMI. Let's take a detailed look at how to identify each category, and what possible measures you can take to help yourself or someone you know.

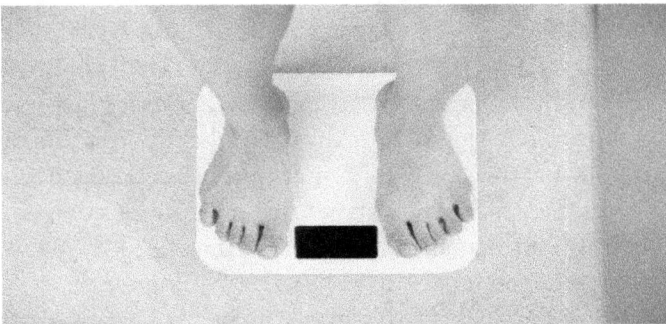

Based on Site of Fat Deposition

By using this method of locating fatty deposits in your body, you will come across two main categories of obesity.

Android Obesity

Android obesity, also known as abdominal obesity, is the category where most of your fat will be found in your upper body area—in the abdomen region. This type of obesity is commonly found in obese men, and in women who have just gotten over their menopause and whose estrogen levels are decreasing. It's highly advised to seek medical help as soon as you notice fat accumulation in your abdominal area and should not be taken lightly because it can affect your metabolism, and how you perform activities in daily life.

Here's how to diagnose if you might have android obesity. While the general BMI is calculated by weight (lb.) over height (ft²); to identify abdominal obesity, you must use your waist circumference as well. The waist circumference of men should not exceed 37 inches, and for women it should not exceed 31.5 inches. Being over these numbers would ideally mean that you have androgenic or abdominal obesity.

There can be many different causes for this type of obesity. First is getting it through your genes. If both your parents have abdominal obesity, then you're 80% more likely to get it yourself, and if it's just one parent, you're 25% more likely to get it. In any case, it's important to be mindful if either of your parents have abdominal obesity and take extra care from the very start. Secondly, you can get this type of obesity from consuming too much food; fluctuations in your hormones; side effects of certain medications; slow metabolism; or even psychological issues.

With this type of obesity, you can expect shortness of breath after a short walk, being tired after waking up, or by doing minimal activity; type 2 diabetes from over consumption of food; arterial hypertension from having constant high blood pressure, and many heart-related issues—including a heart attack, etc.

Possible treatments for this category are to seek medical help and get a diet plan advised and recommended by your doctor. In that case, you must follow and stick to that diet to see weight loss. In addition, you can take up more interest in physical activities. Don't give in to your body weight and sit around watching TV. Instead, join a team for your favorite sport. Rather than watching it, do it. The more active you become, the easier it will be for you to lose that abdominal weight and become fitter again. As a last resort, you can even consider surgical treatment. But only do that when you find none of the diets and physical activities are working and do it only with your doctor's consent. Since surgical treatments can be complicated and expensive, it's best to keep them as your last possible resort.

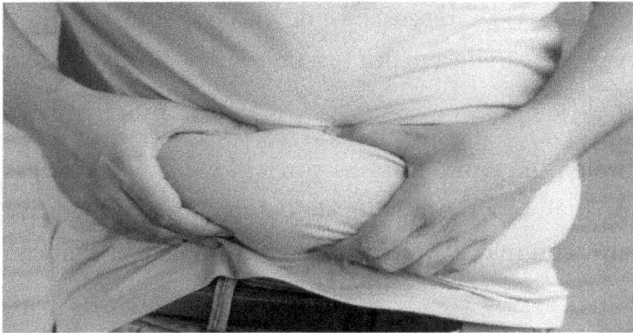

Gynoid Obesity

Typically, it's observed by females where the fat gets deposited over the breasts, hips, and thighs. Gynoid obesity is the abundance of fat in those areas, more so than the normal amount. Gynoid fats develop during and after puberty, getting the body ready to hold and nurture a potential child. These fatty deposits are guided by hormones to keep them under control. However, gynoid obesity occurs when fat accumulates only in these areas resulting in a "pear shape." However, gynoid fat in a durable amount is very vital because it allows for the breasts to produce and supply breastmilk. The gynoid fats in breastmilk are what help the baby's brain and body develop. It's very important to know when gynoid fat turns into obesity, which can then harm the female body rather than benefit it. Gynoid obesity can also be found in men when their fat starts to accumulate in their thighs and buttocks compared to anywhere else.

To diagnose this type of obesity, you need to find the hip-to-waist ratio using their circumferences. If the ratio you get is below 0.80, then you're suffering from gynoid obesity. Obesity of this type can occur for a variety of reasons. If it's genetic, it will most likely be from Bardet-Biedl syndrome and can also be inherited from your parents. But other than these factors, you can also develop gynoid obesity from a lack of exercise. This can also be in the form of working from home full-time due to easy lifestyle choices; stress can also make you obese as well as other mental health issues as discussed in the previous chapter; consumption of fatty foods can be a major reason for developing gynoid obesity.

With this type of obesity, the complications you will face are shortness of breath, sleep apnea, high blood pressure, varicose veins, and digestive problems. Additionally, you may also have tumors from cancer that can be deathly.

Fighting this type of obesity is the hardest of all. You might find it very hard to lose weight and need to work very hard with a fixed routine to reduce fat in the area where gynoid fat is located. You will need to adopt a diet that is very strict and low in calorie count. Snacking becomes taboo when you become obese with this type as you cannot move away from your diet. Along with that, physical activity is a must to get the energy consumption up and burn the fat more. Since gynoid obesity is hard to fight, and requires a lot of dedication, it's advised that people fighting it seek psychological help to ensure no extra stress is caused; you don't develop mental health problems; and you get the motivation needed to fight this obesity.

develop mental health problems; and you get the motivation needed to fight this obesity.

Based on Your BMI

These following categories will help you identify where you fall with the help of your BMI.

Underweight

As mentioned above, your BMI is calculated by dividing your height by your weight. If you get a result of less than 18.5, then you're underweight for your height and size. This means that you must take the necessary steps to gain weight and get to the normal weight category.

Just like being overweight, there are risks and consequences to being underweight as well. While you may not necessarily face all the complications, you might be subject to any of the following: osteoporosis; skin, hair, or teeth complications; weakened immunity; tiredness; anemia; irregular periods in women; premature birth by an underweight pregnant woman; and slow growth are all possibilities.

What caused the issue of being underweight could be family history and genes, a very fast-working metabolism, illness or disease, or mental issues. While the treatment for being underweight is to consume more calories, it's also advised to not dive into fatty foods as they will still harm your body and subject you to different heart conditions.

Normal Healthy Weight

The BMI for this category should be between 18.5 and 24.9. This is the ideal range that every man, woman, and child should fit into. Being 18.4 would be considered as being underweight and being 25 would be considered as being overweight. At this level, you reduce your exposure to many problems and diseases like heart attacks, strokes, cancer, diabetes, body pain, and anemia. All while increasing your self-esteem, having a stronger immune system, and being energetic.

To maintain this level, you must make the correct food choices like consuming the right amounts of vegetables, fruits, meats, carbs, and even fats. It also means being physically active and fit. Whether it's a daily run or playing your favorite sports, it's important to keep the discipline of being fit to remain healthy. Moreover, it's also a healthy practice to stay properly hydrated to reduce issues such as dehydration and feeling tired after a good night's sleep. It's also advisable to keep your alcohol and other substances to a limit, or even better, not consumed at all. Lastly, it's important that you be aware of your weight to keep check whether you're healthy.

Overweight

You start being overweight the minute your BMI exceeds 25 until it reaches 29.9. Being overweight and not controlling it is the first step to obesity. Curbing your weight at this stage is comparatively easier. There are studies that show how you're less at risk when compared to those at the obese stage. However, the risks are expected to be lower and milder, but not zero. Compared with the other levels of obesity, the mortality rate of overweight people is slightly lower at 0.95, while class one obesity is at 1.18 (Flegal et al., 2013).

You may experience similar symptoms to those who are obese but at a milder range. For example, you may get tired after a job, but it won't be as bad as an obese person. You will still be able to run an extra mile if you push yourself, but an obese person may not be able to do even that. You may get high blood pressure and high cholesterol levels, but if you monitor them, they may not be at a dire level and can be brought down by exercise, curbing your food intake, and drinking lots of water.

Class 1—Obesity

When you cannot control your calorie intake, and the amount exceeds the one that burns your fat, the fat starts to accumulate over time drastically increasing your weight. Once your BMI reaches 30 until 34.9, you're in class 1 obesity. You will start to find it hard to exercise and move around with the fat that starts to weigh you down. Aside from consuming food frequently, and not being able to control it, this level can also be reached by excessive amounts of alcohol and other substances including drugs and/or steroids. Moreover, you can get to class 1 obesity with age as the metabolism slows down, and with the intake of high calories, it's not hard to gain weight and not easy to lose it.

Because this is the stage where you're ingesting more calories than are being burned, you need to focus on limiting your intake of calories here. Intermediate fasting diets and keto diets are applicable here because they focus on burning fat to provide energy. The burning of fat can also happen from workouts. This may be harder to do at this stage, but the effort you put in will show in your physical and mental health.

Class 2—Severe Obesity

Severe obesity is when your BMI ranges from 35 to 39.9. This is not a light case of obesity. It can lead to very painful problems and can possibly cause death as well. According to Obesity Class II (n.d.), this class of obesity can lead to high blood pressure, lipid abnormalities, atherosclerosis, vascular degeneration, coronary heart disease, congestive heart failure, stroke, hypoventilation, type 2 diabetes, gallbladder disease, osteoarthritis, colorectal, breast, and uterine cancers.

Along with the health problems, it can also cause severe self-esteem issues as people become more insecure, depressed, and even disgusted with their own bodies. The discrimination faced by the world can also be something you will face at this level of obesity. Diets and eating plans are crucial to helping fight obesity at this stage, along with whatever physical activities you can take on. At this stage, if nothing seems to work, people can also consider surgical removal of fat.

Class 3—Morbid Obesity

Having a BMI of 40 or more along with being 100 pounds over your ideal weight is classified as morbid obesity. Over 24 million adults in the United States are morbidly obese and qualify for the surgical procedure (University Health Care, n.d.).

A simple walk will become a hike, and the health consequences are dire at this level of obesity. From heart diseases to complications with your kidneys, if you have this class of obesity, it's vital to seek medical help immediately, and follow the guidelines provided by them.

Chapter 4:
Diagnose if You're Obese

Now that you know the different types of obesity, and what can cause them, it's important that you know how to diagnose if you have obesity, and how to identify which level or category you fall under. You won't be able to identify which category you fall under by just checking your weight. You need to have much more to be able to correctly identify and seek medical help when you need it. Like it has already been mentioned above, gaining a pound or two doesn't mean that you have obesity. So, let's look at various methods and ways you can use to find out if you are obese and which category you fall under.

Methods of Obesity Screening

There are two types of screening you can do to identify obesity, and they are checking for it yourself or running a test in a diagnostic lab. Let's investigate each aspect in detail.

Self-Screening

Obesity is a serious concern because it's associated with poorer mental health outcomes, reduced quality of life, and one of the leading causes of death in the U.S. and worldwide (CDC, 2020). Therefore, it's important that everyone must know how to self-screen for obesity, know when it's overweight that needs to be thwarted, and know when to seek medical help. Self-screening can be done in two ways: waist measurement and BMI calculations.

Your BMI should ideally range from 18.5 to 24.0 or from the 5th to the 84th percentile. If it exceeds that, then you're considered overweight. But that doesn't always mean that you're obese and are going to suffer health complications. You're only obese if your BMI is over 30 or the 85th percentile or higher. It's only then that you need to seek medical help. You can do it prior to that as well, but it's not as dire as once your BMI reaches the obesity range. Because if not given the proper attention, obesity can reach the morbid stage.

The second step in self-screening is to measure your waist. Your ideal waist measurement should not exceed 37 inches for men and 31.5 inches for women. The increase can result in heart conditions and many more complications. There can be instances where your BMI is in the normal range, but your waist size increases from the measurements above. It's still considered risky for your health, and you should consult medical help. It's advisable that you check your waist measurement at least once every six months or within a year at the most. Obesity and being overweight are especially dangerous if they run in your family or are the result of a disorder or disease.

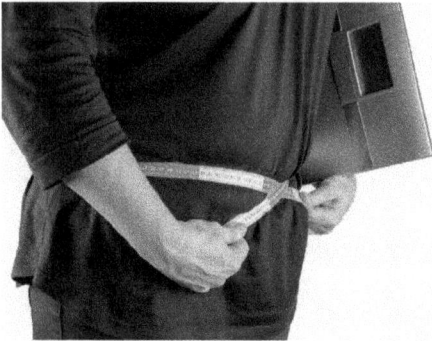

A few other precautions you can take by yourself are keeping up with your health history, any past conditions or screening for other conditions, and doing a body check, measuring your blood pressure, diabetes, height, etc.

Lab Tests

There are multiple tests that can help you identify the severity of obesity.

Thyroid Test

As obesity is one of the consequences when the thyroid hormones fluctuate, it's also important that you get a thyroid test if you see yourself gaining weight very easily. This can help you stop it before it gets any worse. The test requires you to give blood but requires no prior preparation from your side. However, it's important to inform your doctor if you're taking any medications, or if you're suffering from any other disorders.

There are two tests that can help determine if you have thyroid problems. The thyroid-stimulating hormone (TSH) test is done to determine if you have hyperthyroidism or hypothyroidism. If your TSH test results are higher than 4.5 mU/L, then you will experience weight gain as a symptom of hypothyroidism. Now if you find out it's your thyroid fluctuations that cause you to gain weight, you need to take the steps accordingly to resolve the thyroid problem before you can focus on losing weight.

Liver Function Test

This test is needed to diagnose if you have fatty liver disease, which can happen either from too much alcohol consumption or for other reasons. This disease can cause weight gain, and the fat deposits in your liver can also give you type-2 diabetes. It can lead to liver failure and other deadly diseases. Thus, it's extremely important to get it tested. It's again a blood test that you will have to give, and you will have to prepare for it by avoiding eating before as certain foods can affect the tests, compromising the results.

There are many different tests you can do to determine if your liver is damaged. The tests below will help you identify which one to take, and what the normal results should be:

- Alanine transaminase helps you convert the protein into energy. The normal range of results should be from 7 to 55 units per liter (U/L).

- Aspartate transaminase is found in low blood levels and helps metabolize amino acids. The normal result ranges from 8 to 48 U/L.

- Alkaline phosphatase is an enzyme that helps break down proteins. The normal result should range from 40 to 129 U/L.

Fasting Blood Sugar

If you have diabetes or think that you have diabetes, it's important that you follow up on it, and take precautionary measures to keep it under control. Diabetes is a consequence and a cause of obesity. If you don't control what you eat, you may get diabetes and gain weight. Likewise, if you have diabetes, and don't keep it under control, or don't know about it, you can find yourself gaining weight. The most definite way to test for diabetes is the blood sugar test. But for this test, you will need to fast for up to eight hours prior to the test to get the most accurate results. Eating food, even if it contains natural sugar, can alter the results of this test.

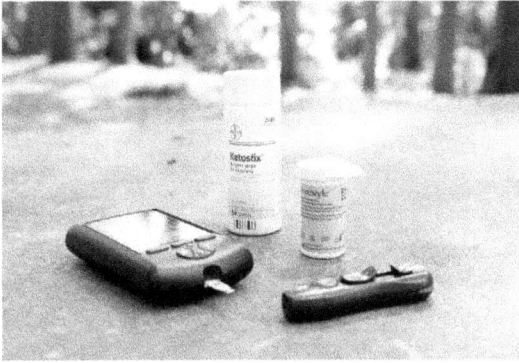

A normal range of results should be from 70–100 mg/dl, and a higher result will make you diabetic. This can also be a reason you gain weight, and no matter the exercise, you may find it hard to lose weight if you don't control your sugar levels in this case.

Cholesterol Test

The cholesterol test will check if you have low, high, or normal cholesterol; levels of triglycerides in your body; and lipoprotein found. The total cholesterol level found in your body should not be more than 200 mg/dl. If it's less than 100 mg/dl, then you have low cholesterol levels. Cholesterol is also a result of obesity, and if you think you're gaining weight, it's better to check your cholesterol levels as high cholesterol leads to heart attacks and strokes.

For this test, you will have to fast for a couple of hours for the most accurate results and will have to provide a blood sample. There are home cholesterol tests available too, but for the most accurate results or to double check, it's better that you get it tested at a medical facility.

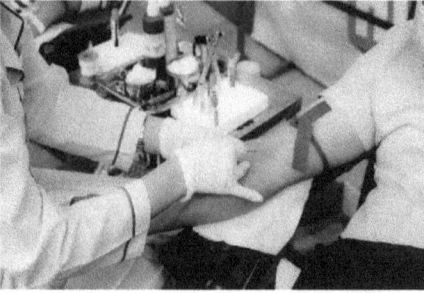

Skinfold Measurement

This is the measurement where your fat will be evaluated and converted into a percentage to compare how much of it is in your body. It's tested on the right side of your body with instruments that can accurately determine the amount of fat found. Some of the areas that are measured are the abdomen, triceps, quadriceps, pectoral area, etc. To calculate the body fat percentage, you must enter the measurements into software (which can be found online as well). However, the accuracy of this test is the lowest as the measurements taken need to be precise, and the room for human error is greater here.

Chapter 5

Major Risk of Heart Attacks and Strokes Owing to Obesity

Even though it has already been highlighted that obesity increases your risk of a heart attack and stroke, which can be deadly, it needs to be taken very seriously. However, Jennifer Logue at the University of Glasgow (n.d.) says, "two new things: obese, middle-aged men have a 60% increased risk of dying from a heart attack than non-obese, middle-aged men, even after we cancel out any of the effects of cholesterol, blood pressure, and other cardiovascular risk factors."

If obesity alone is fatal, then the added factor of heart attacks and strokes is just going to ensure that your life won't be easy and healthy. Instead of spending your time with your friends and family, you will be worrying about hospital bills, and when your next attack could take you out. And that won't be the end of it. You will have to monitor yourself constantly for other disorders, which can take a toll on you mentally, physically, and financially. Before we look at other factors that can increase the risk of heart attacks in an obese person, let us look at who's affected worse and why.

Who's at Greater Risk?

Backed up by results from a study, adults between the ages of 40–59 are at a greater risk of developing heart disease and dying from a heart attack (Khan et al., 2018). As a child, your immunity is stronger, but once you reach this age, your immunity is already weaker, and with the increase in the chances of heart attacks and strokes, your chances of surviving them decrease. If your stroke or attack does not turn out to be deadly, it will take a toll on your mental health. You will have to be extra careful and will gradually be restricted on activities. When you reach old age, you won't be able to move or do the simplest of activities because you have suffered through so much in your 40s and 50s. Moreover, if you have struggled with obesity since childhood, then your immunity tends to weaken faster than compared with normal adults, which will result in you being at greater risk after your 40s of a heart attack or stroke.

Boosters That Escalate the Risk

Let's talk about certain choices that you may make that will add to the risk of you having a heart attack or stroke and make the impact worse, along with suffering from obesity.

Drugs

Drugs are addictive substances that make your heart's condition worse. Even the frequent inclusion of painkillers can cause your heart condition to weaken and make you more prone to suffering from a heart attack or stroke. On top of that, if you're obese, your body is not strong enough to fight back everything at once, much like an overloaded circuit. Thus, your chances of having a heart attack increase and become worse with the use of drugs and being obese.

Stress

To show the impact stress has on dying from a heart attack, let's take the example of Tim Russert. An American TV show journalist and lawyer died at the age of 58 after suffering from a heart attack. His case is vital to prove that stress makes the impact of heart attacks worse because he was diagnosed with obesity and was working toward fighting it. His life expectancy was predicted to be approximately 70 years and above, which made his death shocking to the doctors. It was the amount of stress he took on top of being obese that made his heart attack worse and killed him. According to statistics back in 2008, 40% of people in America used to die after suffering from a heart attack, and that percentage has only grown with the rise in obesity (Elflein, 2022).

So, how does stress make your attacks worse? When a person suffers from an attack, it's due to the bursting of arteries or blockage of blood and oxygen. Stress can also aid in all that raising your heart rate by an abnormal amount, and sometimes, even restricting the oxygen levels, causing the heart attack to be much worse and possibly deadly.

Smoking

Obesity and smoking have a tight relationship. People who are obese and would like to lose weight often tend to start smoking and become addicted. And people who want to quit smoking start gaining weight, which if not handled properly, can lead to obesity. This cycle, even though it looks never-ending, is extremely harmful to anyone involved. Whether you're an obese person smoking, which will cause you severe heart attacks with multiple more problems, or you are a smoker who decided to quit and is gaining weight rapidly, getting diagnosed with obesity and all the problems that come along with it. Obese people who smoke are likely to lose 13 years off their lives in comparison to people of healthy weight and those who do not smoke (Peeters et al., 2003).

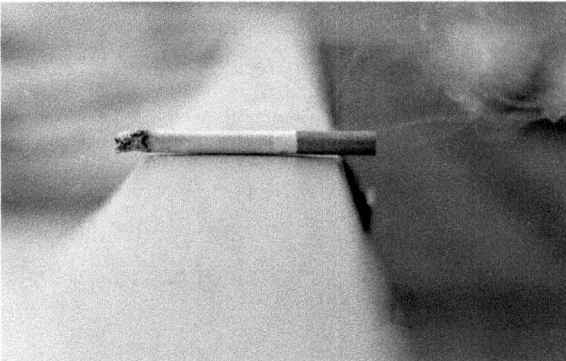

Inactivity

If you're a victim of obesity or once was, being in good shape should always be your top priority. Because if you start exercising and working out, your body will start to fight along with you and help you burn those fats that can increase your chances of a deadly heart attack. Even if you're dieting and cutting down on carbs, you still must exercise and keep your blood flowing at a normal pace. If you're considering surgery to get your fat removed and think you can just relax from now on, you're wrong because the amount of money you will be spending to get rid of excess fat will go to waste as fat can easily accumulate again due to inactivity. Thus, it's very important for you to take your physical activity routines very seriously and stick to them. If not, you're practically begging for heart attacks and strokes to come and kill you.

Diabetes

Being an obese person naturally increases the odds of you getting diabetes. But, if not controlled and monitored properly, diabetes can worsen heart attacks. If you have diabetes, you're twice as likely to have heart disease or a stroke as someone who doesn't have diabetes—and at a younger age; the longer you have diabetes, the more likely you are to have heart disease (CDC, 2020a). Having high blood sugar and letting it get out of control frequently can make your heart weaker and expose you to having heart problems.

Diabetes also contributes to high blood pressure and bad cholesterol levels, which when combined with obesity, can reduce life expectancy, and cause fatal heart conditions. Furthermore, if not a heart attack, then diabetes can make your heart fail. This means that your heart is unable to successfully pump blood, depriving the rest of your body of oxygen and causing other problems. It can also cause you a big hit financially with surgeries and medical procedures to get you out of extreme danger but still not perfectly healthy.

High Cholesterol

High cholesterol is when fat-like deposits block your blood flow from your arteries, which can also result in organ failure by colluding your heart. However, not all cholesterol is bad. But the amount of cholesterol that's needed by the body is produced by your liver. It's the additional cholesterol that's bad for your body, that blocks your veins and arteries. According to Harvard Health Publishing (2014), lowering your cholesterol by 10% can reduce the chances of suffering a heart attack or stroke by almost 30%. If you suffer from cholesterol problems, it's always advisable to steer away from fried foods, red meat, sweets, and even dairy products as much as possible. Cholesterol problems can range from you not having enough HDL, also known as "good cholesterol," and having too much LDL, which is the bad side of cholesterol that carries it through your arteries, creating a blockage for blood flow.

High Triglyceride Levels

Your triglyceride levels basically inform you of the fat that you have stored and not being converted into energy. The difference between cholesterol and triglycerides is that cholesterol is used to create cells and hormones in your body, while triglycerides are used to make energy out of fat. High cholesterol will cause blockage in your veins and arteries, but high levels of triglycerides will cause the hardening of arteries, which can again increase your risk of having a stroke or an attack and can make it affect your body worse. Moreover, it can also cause inflammation in your pancreas. A natural way to help lower your triglyceride levels is by incorporating fish oil into your diet because of the high levels of omega-3 in it.

Hypertension

Hypertension, also known as high blood pressure, can not only increase your chances of a heart attack but also cause many more heart-related problems for you. When the blood flows at a high pressure, the narrow and thin walls of the arteries are weakened and can even burst. The body is made in such a way that the arteries reach every single part, thus, requiring them to be small and flexible, but continuous blood pressure at a high level can easily damage them. This then affects the blood reaching the heart, from there it circulates throughout the body with oxygen and other materials that are required by the body. Not only will your circulation be affected, but your heart might fail, you might have a heart attack or stroke that could kill you, and you might even get a large left lung. A large left lung happens when your heart must work extra hard to pump blood and can cause the muscles of the left chamber of your heart to thicken, further adding to the chances of having a heart attack.

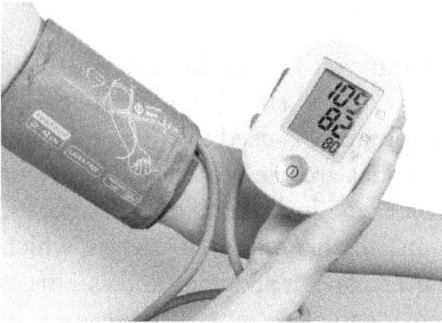

Family History

If you're an obese person with a family history of such or are a person who's not obese but on the overweight side with a family history, you're still prone to having heart attacks and strokes. Because it's in your genes to gain weight easily, you must work extra hard since you're more at risk than a healthy person with healthy parents. You may not be obese, but still find yourself going through the same problems by just being a little over your normal weight. This is because obesity and easy weight gain run in your family, and you need to take extra care—exercise and monitor what you eat more carefully—than a healthy person, or even an overweight person, with no family history of obesity would.

Chapter 6:
Various Health Issues Associated With Obesity

If you're obese, you will not just suffer from one problem or one disorder; you will face many problems in different areas of your body. This is what obesity is. It will affect every part of your life. From your body to your mental health to your social life. It will affect your loved ones and your friends. It will affect your ability to do tasks such as go to work without it being a big deal. It will drain you of your energy and financially as well. That's why it's extremely important, and it has been highlighted before, that you fight obesity at its earliest.

Before you set out to find the correct motivation to help you fight your obesity, you need to be fully aware of the consequences and just how severe they are. Before we move onto the social challenges that you will face with obesity, let's take a deeper look at diseases and disorders that can be a consequence of obesity; how they will have an impact on your life; and treatment options for those that are available.

Cancer

Cancer is one of the many results of obesity, and while cancer doesn't have a cure, we can prevent getting cancer by staying in healthy shape. Obesity can cause 13 different types of cancer, some of which can be truly painful and lead to death. Every 1 in 20 people that get diagnosed with cancer is because of being overweight. If that number doesn't seem daunting enough, then according to a study, 22,800 cases of cancer can be prevented every year in the UK by people living a healthy lifestyle (Bhaskaran et al., 2014).

The fat in your body doesn't just sit and wait; it sends signals and helps cells divide faster and multiply more than the normal amount, leading to cancer. For women, after menopause, the estrogen hormones that are produced by the ovaries can lead to breast and womb cancer. So, elderly women must be careful once they reach menopause because can they naturally gain weight and should also have themselves checked for breast and womb cancer. Moreover, some of the other types of cancers that can affect an obese person are liver, kidney, gallbladder, blood, pancreatic, etc. Not all these cancers will be treatable once diagnosed, which is why it's highly important to know the major side effects of obesity and fight it as soon as you get diagnosed with it before it comes to a point where treatment will not cure the disease, but only be able to decrease it. Pancreatic cancer, as mentioned above, is one of the hardest cancers to treat, and you will be exposed to a lot of pain throughout (Cancer Research UK, 2018).

Additionally, the location of fat in your body can also affect which type of cancer you're most likely to get. For example, if you have abdominal obesity, then you're much more exposed to kidney, esophagus, breast, and bowel cancer. This is theorized to be because the chemicals and signals travel quicker from your belly to these places.

Cardiovascular Diseases

Cardiovascular disease refers to problems with your blood vessels that reach your body parts from the heart and back. Before we investigate the details of cardiovascular disease, let us look at the different types of diseases.

- Cerebrovascular disease happens if there are problems with the vessels that supply blood to your brain.
- Coronary heart disease happens when there is a problem with the vessels supplying blood to your heart.
- Congenital heart disease refers to deformities in the structure of your heart that typically occur at birth.
- Vein thrombosis and pulmonary embolism is when blood clots form in your veins that can start in your legs and move to your heart.
- Rheumatic heart disease indicates that there's damage to your heart valves and muscles.
- Peripheral arterial disease happens if there are problems with the vessels supplying blood to and from the arms and legs.

The most common symptoms of these diseases are usually chest pains, heart attacks, and strokes. But depending on your body type, and how severe the disease is, the symptoms vary from feeling numbness in your arms and legs to feeling nauseous and fatigued frequently.

Treating cardiovascular diseases means having the necessary medicines and getting certain surgeries done. Since it's an issue with your blood vessels and the heart, you must rely on medicines and surgeries. In the event of a stroke, the medications prescribed will be able to calm it down. Because the treatment relies on medicine and medical development, countries with underdeveloped medical facilities face increased death rates due to heart attacks and strokes from cardiovascular diseases. The simplest medicines you can keep ready at your side are beta-blockers, aspirins or painkillers, statins, and angiotensin. Moreover, some surgeries that you may have to consider for cardiovascular diseases are valve repair, heart operations and transplants, angioplasty, and artery bypass.

Reproductive Disorders

Obesity affecting the reproductive system is not just for females but can also be seen in males. From infertility to birth-related problems, obesity does make many disorders worse. However, it's seen mostly in females in terms of infertility. In a study conducted by the Reproductive Medicine Unit at the University of Adelaide in Australia (n.d.), it was found that out of 5,000 women who were infertile, 40% had their BMI above the normal weight range, and 17% of those were overweight. Such a high number from just one disease is a major deal and needs to be taken seriously.

Weight gain in women also affects their ovulation rates. This is proved in a study conducted at Queen Elizabeth Hospital in Australia where women who were overweight and had their ovulation patterns recorded, drastically changed after losing over 10 pounds. Moreover, more than half of the women were able to achieve pregnancy (Australian Institute of Health and Welfare, 2019). But obesity just does not create infertility; there are many women who are obese or overweight and have achieved pregnancy and given birth successfully too. However, the complications that may arise make the pregnancy journey for the mother hard and extremely painful. For example, obesity may create gestational problems where you may not deliver normally and would have to choose the cesarean method. That method can then create many more complications should you get pregnant again.

Obesity in men affects their semen production and ejaculation rates. Although men's reproductive systems are not affected as much as the reproductive systems of females, that does not reduce the impact. There can be instances where men can be sub fertile, and this can affect pregnancy rates in women.

Asthma

Obesity is going to increase your chances of getting asthma, and if you already have asthma, then obesity is going to make it worse. This is very serious for people who already have asthma and are obese too. Because obesity can cause a lot of shortness of breath, people who have asthma already start getting severe attacks and need to head to the hospital frequently or buy equipment and keep it handy in case they get an asthma attack.

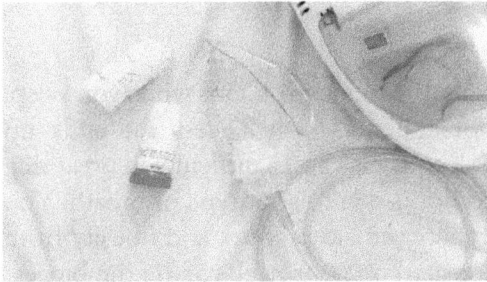

According to the CDC (2019), there are more asthmatic people who are also obese than there are asthmatic people who are healthy. Obesity causes asthma and shortness of breath because the fat in your body causes inflammation around your lungs, restricting your airway. This makes it hard to breathe after small amounts of exercise too. Obesity also makes patients' bodies irresponsive to corticosteroids that are prescribed to asthmatic people who are not obese. Since then, obese patients become less responsive to medication, their hospital visits increase, and they start to experience severe asthmatic attacks.

Moreover, the symptoms are made worse by environmental factors and family history that one cannot do anything about immediately. Obese people living in a city with heavy pollution and smoke will have severe attacks of asthma compared to obese people living somewhere with less pollution and more fresh air.

To help reduce the severity and frequency of attacks, it's important to lose weight and get physically active. It will be hard in the beginning, but you can overcome it with the right preparation and the proper medical equipment by your side in case you suffer an attack. You can also seek medical help and follow through with the medication you get prescribed, even if you think there's no improvement to be seen. If you have suffered from asthma since birth, and obesity has just come to you, then losing your weight is vital for you to not suffer from severe and often attacks of asthma.

Sleep Apnea

Sleep apnea is when you suffer from breathing problems when you sleep. Obesity makes sleep apnea worse because the excess fat ends up blocking your airways while you sleep. This causes difficulty in breathing and can have you wake up at odd hours due to shortness of breath. You can also identify the relationship between sleep apnea and obesity from your neck measurement. Fat deposited on your neck can be the biggest reason for sleep apnea. The acceptable neck circumference is 17 inches for men and 16 inches for women. The more the number increases, the worse your sleep apnea will get. Sleep apnea is more commonly found in men than women and is found more in people with a higher BMI.

Symptoms of sleep apnea include daytime sleeping, snoring at night, and waking up frequently during the night. Sleep apnea also increases your chances of a heart attack or stroke.

You can treat your sleep apnea by using a continuous positive airway pressure (CPAP). This machine can be set beside at night. You can put this mask on for a better night's sleep. But this machine can be a burden because it needs to stay on to work, which would restrict your movements while sleeping, making you uncomfortable. It would also be needed if you're napping to be able to sleep without sleep apnea. Many people with sleep apnea don't get accustomed to the machine. An alternative to this option is to lose weight. Those who suffer from obesity and sleep apnea should try to lose weight as it effectively helps with their sleep apnea. You can consult the medical facilities to help you with the most effective way for you to lose weight. Losing even the smallest amount of weight will show great improvement in your sleep apnea. Ten percent weight loss will help your sleep apnea by 20% (Kucera, 2018).

Alzheimer's Disease

Alzheimer's is getting more common in aged people. But it can also happen from obesity. Obesity may not directly cause Alzheimer's, but it affects your insulin resistance, which plays a great role in Alzheimer's. Insulin resistance can decrease your brain volume through decreasing glucose metabolism in your brain and making insulin in your brain dysfunctional. A higher BMI can also decrease white matter, which affects your learning abilities; it can decrease cognitive abilities; and it can increase your chances of getting Alzheimer's. Moreover, obesity in your 40s–60s can also increase your chances of getting dementia.

If you're an obese person and get Alzheimer's, then you may experience natural weight loss. This could be due to repeating tasks or forgetting tasks. For example, you could increase physical activity by repeating tasks and forgetting to eat, reducing your weight. Brock University in Canada conducted a study where they concluded that high fat and sugar diets have increased the occurrence of Alzheimer's in old people (Baranowski et al., 2018). Your diet matters if you have obesity, and it's important that even if you don't have obesity, you watch what you eat and ensure high sugar and fat levels are not part of your diet daily.

Alzheimer's cannot be cured, but there are treatments out there that can help slow the progression of the disease by managing behavioral changes and maintaining the functionality of your brain. Which is why it's vital that when you get diagnosed with obesity, you immediately work hard to fight it. The earlier you start, the better your chances of escaping Alzheimer's in your old age become. Make sure your diet is healthy and does not contain much sugar and fat and keep up your physical activity. The better your health, the better your brain will become.

Type-2 Diabetes

Obesity is one of the major reasons people get type-2 diabetes. Obese or overweight people account for 90% of type-2 diabetics (Vitagene, 2018). If you're obese, it's extremely likely that you will be a diabetic, which is why controlling your diet is important to make sure your diabetes stays under control and doesn't get out of hand.

Obesity increases fatty-acid levels and inflammation that leads to insulin resistance that can lead to type-2 diabetes. Diabetes type-2 is also known as non-insulin-dependent diabetes. People with type-2 diabetes can produce a little insulin, but it's often insufficient, or the body's cells don't respond to it. Because of insulin resistance glucose accumulates in the body resulting in high blood sugar. Type-2 diabetes symptoms include frequent increased thirst, increased hunger, urination, fatigue, and dehydration.

Diabetes type-2 can lead to vision problems, nerve damage, infections, heart problems, high blood pressure, mental health problems, ketoacidosis, and stroke (Vitagene, 2018). Because type-2 diabetes is associated with being overweight, treatment for type-2 diabetes frequently focuses on diet and exercise. Medications can also assist the body in making better use of its own insulin. People may also need insulin injections to bring their blood sugar levels back to normal. But on a positive note, type-2 diabetes is highly treatable, but requires dedication and hard work from your side. Once you learn to control your temptations, you will be able to control your diabetes, lose weight, and live life as a healthy person. Even after you do so, you cannot become entirely carefree as you will still have to keep monitoring your weight and sugar to ensure you have not relapsed.

Acanthosis Nigricans (AN)

A skin disorder that's seen commonly in people who suffer from obesity and diabetes. When your body develops insulin resistance, it can lead to your skin forming hyperpigmentation in areas near your neck, palms, reproductive parts, knees, elbows, etc. This is also known as velvet skin disease because the hyperpigmentation causes your skin to have dark patches and form a velvety texture in these areas. When your body develops insulin resistance, it can no longer use the hormone, and insulin in your bloodstream flows in huge amounts. Apart from obesity and diabetes, this can also be hereditary, due to medications, or the aftereffects of other disorders.

In the case of obesity, adipose tissue deposition in the body causes the release of various cytokines, which can end up causing insulin resistance. Obesity-related AN is much more common among adults in patients weighing nearly twice their body weight. Symptoms you may feel are itching, bad odor, and skin tags.

There are home remedies that you can try out to treat acanthosis nigricans. Let's look at them below.

- Coconut wash in the affected areas.
- Orange or oatmeal scrub—it helps bleach the affected areas.
- A lemon and honey mask that helps reduce dark patches on your body and leaves behind moisturized skin.
- Apple aloe vera is frequently used where you find velvet patches.
- Ayurvedic treatments combined with coconut oil.

Other than home remedies, here are some treatments you can consider:

- Vitamin A retinoids, which come in the form of oils and creams, help exfoliate the skin that's affected by hyperpigmentation.
- Metformin, which treats type-2 diabetes, can help treat the cause of your velvet spots.
- Eating foods like bitter gourd, garlic, banana stem, cinnamon, turmeric, ginger, and giloy.
- Avoid foods that are oily and processed.
- Exercise regularly and use proper sunscreen when out in the sun.

Chapter 7:
Social Challenges Related to Obesity

Obesity is not just going to invade your physical lifestyle, it's going to invade your social life, introducing you to various problems that you will face—whether you're in high school, university, or working. It will not stop there. In fact, it will also cause you problems with your friends, family, and co-workers. The impact obesity can have on your social life can sometimes lead to many more psychological problems that then also affect your physical health. Your motivation in life can be deeply impacted to the point that you don't even feel like getting out of bed. You may feel ashamed of your body, and with the addition of social challenges, you may not want to get healthier and would rather just accept it as your fate.

It's important that you remember, despite the social challenges that you face, to rise and work hard to fight obesity. You may not always have supporters in the form of your family or friends, but it's important to find motivation in the fact that you need to be healthy to live a long life. And if things become too difficult, and you become demotivated frequently, you can always reach out to people who are willing to show you the support you require to get back in shape. Let's investigate some of the social challenges an obese person faces, and let's also look at some ways to overcome them.

Being Discriminated and Mocked

There is discrimination in many parts of the world today, and people are taking notice of it. People face discrimination based on their gender, race, and culture, but no one seems to emphasize the fact that people face weight discrimination. It's not always intentional; there's also unintentional discrimination when it comes to weight. But before we investigate that, let's look at the results of this study that proves how people who are obese are looked at as lazy, unstable, and lacking self-discipline (Puhl & Brownell, 2001). This is a part of your life that you will have to fight people for. You need to push past the description and work hard to achieve your goal of losing weight and leading a healthy lifestyle. Moreover, discrimination leads to obese people receiving lower wages and being isolated in workplace meetings (Puhl & Brownell, 2001).

Moving onto unintentional discrimination, there will be instances where you will be left out because of your disorder. It doesn't mean it's anything personal, but since obesity limits your activity boundaries, you may be left out. For children, it can be in the form of being left out of races; for adults, it can be in the form of not being able to get on certain roller-coaster rides with your friends or family. Instead of being offended by it and doing nothing, you should work toward being a healthy weight so your restrictions lift, and you won't be judged based on your weight.

Along with getting discriminated against, you may also encounter instances where you are mocked. It could be anywhere from your workplace to your home. It can be with your friends or even with your family. There are people who won't know how sensitive this issue is, or what you are going through and will throw nasty comments at you discreetly or directly. But it's upon you to rise above that, not let their comments drag you down, and build such strong motivation that you won't break with these comments and continue achieving your goal.

Low Quality of Living

When you have obesity, you are lowering your quality of life. This is because of the many restrictions that get placed on you when you gain weight. You may not be able to do activities that you once loved, you might be judged while doing them, or you just won't have the confidence to do them. For example, you may not be able to play the same sports, pursue selective hobbies, and be able to loosen up yourself because you will have to keep a constant check on your weight and all the other problems. It can also affect your love life. Aside from all the health complications that you will face, you will also face difficulty in finding someone, doing activities with them, and even performing sexually.

You will not be able to perform many activities the same as a healthy person would. That can be off-putting. Even when doing physical exercise, you may start to notice others being better at it and get demotivated that you can't do the same. You might see someone your same age doing things freely that you would not be able to do with the same level of easiness. This is what lowers your quality of life. You won't be able to enjoy much unless you do something about obesity. You will face difficulty while traveling, commuting to places, enjoying a night out, achieving a task at work, and much more. You will find that because of your weight, you get left behind in different aspects of your life.

Poor Relationships With People

When you struggle with obesity, you will also struggle to maintain relationships with people. You may find yourself in uncomfortable situations, and even if you try to get past it, you will always face that effort in relationships that healthy people don't notice. Your relationship with your family will change because they may be worried about you and constantly be behind your back trying to lose weight. If that's not the case, then it might change with them because they torment you and exclude you because of your weight. In any case, your relationship with your family members is going to change in one way or another.

Moreover, it will also affect your relationship with your friends. They might not be able to fully relate to what you're going through, which can create awkwardness in your relationship—no matter how supportive they are—and that can lead to you wanting to isolate yourself from them more often. Additionally, it can also change because now friends will have to consider doing activities that won't add any additional harm to your body. For instance, you all may not be able to hang out at bars or your favorite restaurants frequently; they also won't be able to do activities that restrict you like certain sports or adventurous activities.

Lastly, it can also affect your love life. Your bond that you have with someone can break when they must live with the burden of helping you lose weight. Furthermore, the medical problems you suffer will also affect them psychologically because seeing your loved ones not enjoying life is not the most comforting feeling. Seeing you overburdened with obesity and how it impacts your life also has an impact on their life. To sum up, your relationships will not be the same once you suffer from obesity, and while they may become stronger in some cases, for the most part, you're going to form poor relationships.

Difficulty Finding Clothes Your Size

When you see yourself gaining weight, you will not be able to find your size of clothes everywhere. You will have to go to specific shops, which can limit your closet. You will not be able to get everything you might see and like because it won't be in your size. Moreover, you might want to wear oversized clothes, so you can be a little less self-conscious of your physical appearance. In today's world, there are many industries opening where you can find plus-size clothing or dedicated sections in many stores, but they won't always showcase clothes that you may like. This means you'll have to settle for what's available rather than what you want.

Furthermore, you may also find great difficulty in finding certain types of clothing. For example, sportswear. When you fight obesity, and start engaging in more physical activities, you will need clothes that are both appropriate and comfortable which can be hard to find. Even if you find shoes in your size, you may not feel comfortable in them, and that can also be a great loss of motivation. Another example is swimwear. Much of that industry promotes suits that either are skin-tight or can be extremely exposing. However, swimming and water activities are a great way to lose weight, but you might have trouble finding swimwear that's your size and makes you comfortable and confident while wearing it.

This may not be applicable to all, but sometimes when shopping for plus-size clothes, it can be embarrassing. Especially, if you go shopping with your partner or friends, and the shops they like and shop at may not have the clothes you like available in your size. Overall, in many areas of your shopping life, especially clothes, you will find difficulty finding something that you like and are comfortable in.

Difficulty While Traveling

As an obese person, you will have difficulty traveling by many modes of transportation; you will have difficulty traveling for short or long distances; and you will have difficulty before, during, and after traveling. Let us have a deeper look into how obesity is going to make travel an issue.

When you decide to travel, you will have to take certain precautions and considerations, especially if you're traveling internationally. Air travel, as such, puts you in a dangerous situation, but traveling to a country that doesn't offer certain surgeries related to obesity in case of an emergency, becomes highly dangerous for you to visit. On top of that, you may also be uncomfortable traveling on an airplane because of the restricted seat option, and it can get embarrassing in certain situations too. Weight bias can be unpredictable in passengers, and while some may be more understanding of your situation, some may refuse to accommodate you. Air travel is not just a social challenge but is also risky for your health, which is why you should consult a medical authority about the risk and complications and then analyze the precautions you can take.

Even when it's not air travel and is a car-ride with family or friends, you will have to keep in mind your weight and body size when it comes to accommodation, and that can cause unintentional discrimination towards you. You can't blame them because they're thinking about everything and making sure you're comfortable. This can make road trips super uncomfortable for you because you will be confined to the car for a long period of time with very little to no space for movement. This can also apply when you're on a bus journey or on a train. Also, if you are driving, special adjustments will be needed to your seat so your movements don't get restricted, which can be extremely dangerous.

Chapter 8:
Being Obese—a Psychological Trauma

After looking at the various health issues and social challenges, let us also understand how obesity creates psychological trauma that will haunt you very late in life. All the health issues also have an impact on our mental health, and while we focus on treatment to make our physical health better, we forget about our mental health, which then makes us depressed and sad in life even after being healthy physically. You may feel as though life is not worth living and can also suffer from self-harm and suicidal thoughts. Your mental health needs to be given priority as much as you take care of your physical health. If you're not mentally stable or happy, your physical health won't matter much.

Obesity also leaves its imprint on your mental health in the form of depression, mental disorders, stress, anxiety, and much more. We will investigate the psychological impact obesity has on your health to help you prioritize your mental health too, which can also provide a better motivator to get fit physically and fight obesity. You may not feel the impacts of obesity on your mental health, but if you simply ignore them, or refuse to help your mental state, then it's just going to dig its roots deeper.

Eating Disorders

The most common disorder related to obesity is the binge-eating disorder. This disorder can cause you to eat and eat until you can no longer move. It doesn't happen with unhealthy foods only, but with all types of food. Any food in large quantities is not good and should be controlled. People with obesity most often find it difficult to lose weight because of this disorder where they cannot stop eating. And after they binge eat, they get overwhelmed with a sense of guilt and disgust. This can lead many people to seek alternative and unhealthy routes to lose weight. For instance, someone who has a binge eating disorder and is obese may resort to tobacco or induced vomiting to lose weight. This has many health implications and has mental health problems associated with it.

On the other hand, when people start to fight obesity because they're weight-conscious, and worried about their physical appearance, they often tend to take the easy and unhealthy way out. That means they don't overeat, they barely eat. They starve themselves until they lose weight. This habit can cause anorexia, which is extremely dangerous. They will then find themselves going to all extremes just to lose weight, and they will think they're getting healthier, but instead they're harming their body in many ways. If you develop anorexia, it will require a lot of dedication and discipline to start eating healthy food at the appropriate times. Anorexia is the opposite of obesity, which can be an impact of obesity and is equally harmful to your health. Harvard Health Publishing (2014) published certain symptoms that you can track to see if you might suffer from anorexia. They mention that frequently skipping meals, intense exercise, feeling cold suddenly, lack of energy, wanting to be perfect, and continuous weight loss are the symptoms most anorexic people feel. If you're not sure if you have anorexia, and are experiencing some of the symptoms above, then seek medical help, especially if you suffer from obesity.

Depression

When you're obese, the fat cells in your body cause brain inflammation. This happens because of the signal that the fat cells send to your brain. According to a study conducted, people who are obese are 55% more likely to suffer from depression than normal-weight people do (Luppino et al., 2010). Moreover, when you're obese, you also face a lot of social challenges, as discussed in the previous chapter, and that, along with the health problems, can really put someone off. People find it hard to be content with their lives and tend to isolate themselves from the world, which can also lead to depression.

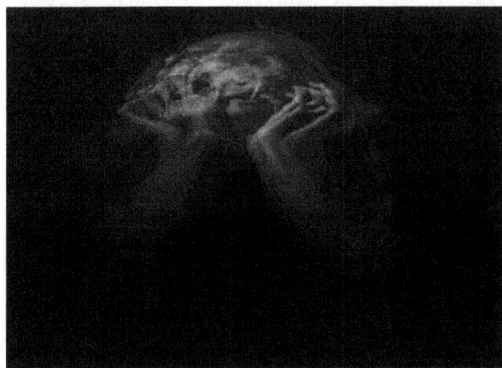

If you find yourself depressed, then it's important that you seek out help, along with working toward losing weight. You will have to give others the benefit of the doubt that they won't always discriminate against you because of your weight and start doing things that make you happy. It's advisable to seek professional help as they can cater to your needs and assist you in just the way you need. Going out to exercise or doing it at home is something you can do on your own, but if you're depressed, then you won't even feel like getting out of bed. Which is why it's completely acceptable to seek help from a friend or to seek professional help. Once you help your depression, losing weight will become much easier than it looks with depression.

Stress and Anxiety

Anxiety affects obese people by 30% more than it does healthy people (CDC, 2008). However, obesity doesn't directly have an impact on anxiety levels, but it does affect your mental health which can lead to anxiety. Similarly, to stress, obesity can create stressful situations when hanging out with people or when in a workplace environment. Because of obesity, your stress levels can increase from what they were before, and you will feel stressed more frequently. Having an abundance of fat cells in your body generates a negative impact on your hormones which can make your emotions all over the place. You may feel stressed to an extreme level even when the situation itself is not that stressful or serious. You will then have to focus more on your mental health, with such high levels of stress and anxiety, than on losing weight and becoming physically healthier.

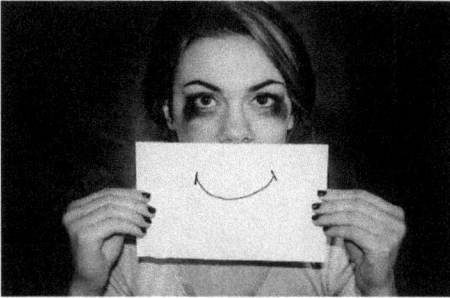

Low Self-Esteem and Self-Confidence

In a study conducted, it was found that people with obesity had lower self-esteem than those who were of normal weight (Schwimmer et al.,

2003). Low self-esteem may result from obesity. You could lose confidence due to being obese. You could face discrimination, mockery, and jokes about your extreme weight. This might have an impact on you by diminishing your confidence which would then lower your self-esteem. You may start to overeat which contributes to more weight gain. The two situations can be viewed as an obesity-esteem cycle that has a cascading effect on a person's health, quality of life, and relationships with others (Lau, 2003).

Dissatisfaction for Self

Self-dissatisfaction causes a person to develop negative thoughts and feelings about their body and the way they look. Obesity can add to that factor because excess fat can lower your self-esteem and make you feel those negative thoughts and emotions for yourself. You may perceive your ideal body image in one way, but with obesity, it can alter that image and make you lose hope in getting fit. On the other hand, it can lead to people using dangerous alternatives, putting their health at risk while still causing dissatisfaction. Some of the extreme measures can include self-harm or using drugs and starvation to lose weight and look appealing.

Chapter   9:
Financial   Expenses   Associated
With Obesity

Treating obesity is not cheap, and if you don't take care, you might find
yourself stuck with financial issues and debts that can add to your mental
health issues. The total cost of obesity rises by up to $122 billion annually
(Tsai et al., 2010). Obesity can take a toll on your savings, can delay your
retirement, and can also put you into heavy financial debt. Not only will
medical costs drain your bank account, but so will a slew of other
expenses. Let us look at some of the costs you will have to prepare for
with obesity and to fight it.

Expenses on Treatments

When seeking medical treatments for obesity, you will find yourself
approaching counseling, medication, or surgery. Each comes with a cost
that will empty your pockets. To take weight-loss counseling, you will
have to pay a fee regularly. Similarly, medication for the complications
that obesity causes will cost a lot. In research conducted, it was found
out that one of the most common results of obesity is getting diagnosed
with type-2 diabetes, and as we have discussed, diabetes cannot be cured
but controlled. The controls require purchasing medicine and
equipment. In the study, it was found that the annual cost of diabetes
treatment in 2017 was $327 billion (CDC, 2020). Furthermore, when you
consider surgery, it may be a one-time expense, but the cost can empty
your savings account or put you in debt. On average, weight loss surgery
can cost you up to $15,000–25,000 (National Institute of Diabetes,
Digestive, and Kidney Diseases, 2019).

When compared with a healthy-weight person, an obese person spends
more than twice as much on medical costs annually. As mentioned in the

previous chapters, obesity is not just a single strand of worry but comes looped within many other complications. Each of them has its own treatment measures and costs that are billed separately.

Purchasing Plus-Size Clothes

It's significantly seen that plus-size clothing costs more than the normal ones and that's not without reason. When creating plus-size clothing, it's created according to demand and is not mass produced. Moreover, the fabric used will be more in quantity than compared with normal-sized clothing that can lead to it costing more. Also, certain types of clothing are not manufactured much in plus-size, and that requires further alterations adding to the cost of extra labor and machinery that makes plus-size clothing more expensive. So, an obese person would have to spend more on necessities, like clothes, than a normal person would.

Costly Eating Habits

When diagnosed with obesity, it means that you're consuming more calories than the ideal intake, which causes them to accumulate as fatty deposits, so they don't get burned off. So, spending more money on foods to satisfy hunger, even though they're cheap, will add up your food costs as you increase the amount of food you consume resulting in obesity. Even if you start fighting obesity, and going on diets, your food costs will not go down dramatically.

One would think that when treating obesity, the cost of food would come down, but it doesn't. Sure, you will be cutting down on your calories, and that would lower the quantity of food you purchase and consume, but your dietary restriction will cut out all the fried, oily, and fast foods that are cheaper in comparison with the healthy and organic food that you will be advised to eat instead. This means your food costs will also increase. If you rely solely on fast foods, or cheaper foods that are generally unhealthy, your food expenses will rise because of obesity.

Low Productivity = Low Earnings

When you suffer from obesity, your capacity to sit in one position or to think for a long time will be affected. You will get tired very easily; you will find it hard to concentrate and focus for long periods; and you will find it hard to come up with effective solutions in the workplace. Seeing your work deteriorate can either result in no promotion or losing your current promotion. This can also take a toll on your financial status because you will start to spend more than you earn.

Chapter 10

Effective Treatments for Obesity

To treat obesity is not just cutting out calories. You will need to do a lot more to help treat obesity. Because it's such an extreme case, it needs proper attention and medical help to treat it. And treatment just doesn't mean getting surgery; there are many options that you can opt for that will help you treat obesity. Medical-nutrition therapy, hypnotherapy, behavioral therapy, diet therapy, pharmacotherapy, and surgery are among the options. Let us investigate these various options in detail below.

Medical-Nutrition Therapy

Medical-nutrition therapy is used to help you lose weight constantly and in a healthy way that's advised to you by a nutritionist or a dietician. If you follow the plans, and restrictions set out for you, then you should be able to lose 1–1.5 pounds every week. This is a healthy and medically approved way to lose weight. The diet will vary from person to person, and if you stick to it, then weight loss should become easier for you. This form of therapy also helps you with all the complications that happen due to obesity. It will help you control your diabetes, blood pressure, sleep apnea, and strokes.

However, it's important that you follow and stick to the plan provided by the dietician as they will give you the right plan to ensure you lose weight at a healthy rate and don't lose too much weight at once. They will also help you lose the right amount of fat and make sure you won't lose too much muscle mass. If you deter from the plan, and eat more than what's given, then your weight loss will be affected, and you might see yourself losing weight slowly or gaining weight instead. Moreover, if you eat less than what's provided, you will lose weight faster, but you will also be at risk of many health complications.

When you seek this therapy, you will have to keep a journal of your eating habits before a dietician prescribes you a diet that will help you lose fat but will also give you the right amount of energy needed for the day. You will have to keep track of your calories and might have to give up some foods for the healthier option.

Behavioral Therapy

Behavioral therapy helps you change your eating and exercise habits that will in turn help you lose weight. With the help of a therapist, and the support of a group, you will get enough motivation and help to change your lifestyle choices. You will start to watch how much you eat, exercise more often, and set goals that start to become achievable. Before jumping into surgeries and intense medication, your doctor may first ask you to try behavioral therapy unless you suffer from morbid obesity. An added benefit of this therapy is that you can try it with a group suffering from obesity, and you can gain motivation together to lose weight by changing your lifestyle choices. Moreover, once your lifestyle choices become better, they will become your new routine that will help you keep your fitness level the same even after overcoming obesity.

However, when opting for behavioral therapy, many may find it insignificant to lose much weight. You may find yourself not achieving your weight-loss goal, and that could be because the reason for your obesity is not lifestyle choices but family history. Which is why it's important to know the cause of your obesity and use treatments accordingly with the help of medical professionals.

To start with this therapy, you will have to keep a food journal before your first appointment. It's important that you're honest, so the professional can advise you on a plan accordingly to help you lose weight consistently. You will be asked to make small changes in your lifestyle that will help you lose weight, and soon those small changes, over a period, will entirely change your lifestyle to promote weight loss. Lastly, it's important that you remember to meet with your therapist at least two more times after your session comes to an end to ensure that your old habits aren't returning.

Hypnotherapy

Using the help of repetition and mental imagery, therapists can use the hypnotherapy method to bring you into a state of relaxation that can help you change your habits and behaviors. This type of therapy is used not only to help obese patients, but also to change a variety of negative behaviors, emotions, and habits. For instance, it's also used to help people stop smoking. Similarly, it can help you change your habits that have become the cause of obesity. In a study within a controlled environment, 60 participants were tried for hypnotherapy and given diets to follow that helped all of them lose 2–3 pounds within 3 months (Stradling et al., 1998). However, for an obese person, the amount of weight loss within this time limit is not much. In fact, they need to lose as much weight as is healthily possible. But hypnotherapy is successful in helping people retain new eating habits that can help if you find yourself having a "cheat day" every other day.

If you decide to use hypnotherapy, to help you maintain your habits, you will be required to meet with a therapist who will review your goals and get you on the same page about how hypnotherapy works. They will then help you relax by speaking in a soothing voice that will make you feel safe. They will then talk about various eating habits and exercises that you can incorporate into your life that will help you down the road to a healthy life. They may also repeat the statements to get the best results. At the end, they will bring you out of hypnosis.

Hypnotherapy will leave you in a more relaxed state of mind if nothing else and will help you realize the importance of losing that excess weight. However, there are also risks involved in this form of therapy, which are headaches, false-memory creation, drowsiness from imagery, and dizziness.

Diet Therapy

It's pretty much in the name of what you can expect from this therapy. You will be asked to follow a certain type of diet according to your BMI and how your goals are set to lose weight. A major cause of obesity is an unhealthy diet, and getting a diet prepared to suit your individual needs is a very important step toward fighting obesity. For obesity, you will be advised to follow a diet that asks you to strictly cut down on your calories, and not just that, it should be lower than the calories that are burned to see effective weight loss. But just doing that on your own can also lead to cases of starvation and malnutrition. Which is why it's important that you consult the proper professionals to develop a diet that will help you lose weight, and at the same time, give you enough energy to perform activities throughout the day without overeating. This form of therapy also helps with other diseases like constipation, ulcers, anemia, diabetes, and much more.

It's highly advisable that before you start diet therapy, you get a health checkup done. This will help the dietitian prepare a diet keeping in mind any other complications that you may have and your BMI. For instance, if you also suffer from diabetes, then your sugar will be cut down as well, but if you don't, the dietician might add a little room for you in terms of consuming sugar. If the dietician has all the information, they will be able to produce a diet that will suit you the best and will show results of weight loss consistently.

Pharmacotherapy

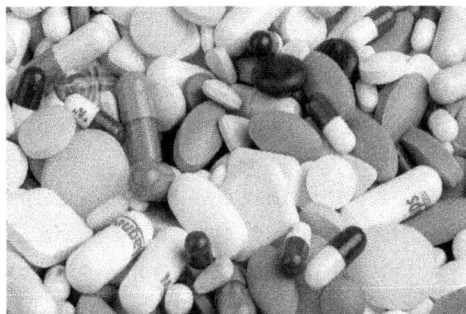

This form of therapy relies on drugs to aid in helping treat obesity. For obesity, there are certain medicines you may be prescribed, and it's important to know why you're prescribed that drug and what risks and benefits are involved. Let's look at the different types of pharmacotherapies used to help treat obese people.

Phentermine

This drug helps you lose your appetite, and when dealing with obesity, can be used with a proper diet and exercise to prevent overeating. If you suffer from obesity, high cholesterol, or high blood pressure, then you will be more likely to be prescribed this drug. However, it's strictly prohibited that you don't consume this drug if you're breastfeeding or pregnant. Because if you consume this drug while pregnant, it can harm the unborn baby, so even if you're obese during pregnancy, it's advisable that you wait until after birth, and then approach healthier ways to lose weight. Moreover, if you suffer from heart disease, thyroid disease, or have a history of drug addiction, then it's suggested that you don't consume this drug. Lastly, don't overuse this drug more than prescribed, and don't miss out on taking it at the prescribed time.

Orlistat

Orlistat is a drug that will help prevent the fat you consume from being absorbed by your body. While it's a drug that helps you lose weight, it mostly focuses on preventing additional weight from being gained. So, when you use this medicine, you must also eat fewer calories in your daily diet and exercise more. Similar warnings should be kept in mind when consuming this drug if you're pregnant or breastfeeding. Moreover, if you have had organ surgery, then it's advisable that you don't take this medicine as a resort to losing weight. If your diet is high in fat—which won't be likely if you are getting your obesity treated—don't resort to this drug as it can have side effects on your stomach and intestines. And it's vital that you treat the medication as an important part of your treatment, but if you stop following the diet or quit exercising, then you won't be able to see effective results and may face side effects instead.

When prescribed orlistat, make sure you follow the instructions on the prescription, and don't miss out on any dosage times or take more to see faster weight loss; that will not happen. If you face any confusion, it's always better to consult your doctor than decide for yourself because if it's not followed properly, then you will have to face the effects of it as well. Additionally, if you miss out on a meal with fat, then you will have to skip taking this drug (confirm with your doctor). Lastly, since orlistat stops the absorption of fat, it can also influence other vitamins and minerals which is why you might have to take supplements for them.

Lorcaserin

Lorcaserin affects the signals in your brain that control your appetite. This, along with a proper diet and exercise, can show significant amounts of weight loss. When taking this medication, it's important that you remember to do it by prescription from your doctor because if not, you may face severe side effects. For instance, lorcaserin does have many side effects if taken with certain other medicines. It can also trigger an allergic reaction, so it's important that you test it first before incorporating it into your daily routine. This tablet should only be swallowed whole, not crushed, or chewed. Lastly, avoid any strenuous activity, like swimming, right after you take this medication.

Liraglutide

While this drug is used to control blood sugar levels in children and adults, a brand of liraglutide, Saxenda, is used to help people lose weight. This medicine is prescribed for adults if you have a BMI greater than 30, and for children who are 12 and weigh over 132 pounds. It works by decreasing your appetite and needs to be taken along with a diet and regular exercise. Another brand of liraglutide, the one used to treat type-2 diabetes, should not be taken simultaneously. Moreover, if you have a thyroid history or suffer from it, you should not take this drug to deal with your obesity. This drug is injected and should be injected as soon as you prepare it. There can be side effects that should be dealt with immediately or can become severe.

Dexfenfluramine

This drug was approved by the United States for its weight loss effect, but can, however, have cardiovascular side effects that resulted in it being discontinued as of September 15, 1997. One of the side effects was pulmonary hypertension as an article published on Drugs.com states that, "Four particular case reports describe that women between the ages of 26 and 46 who had been taking dexfenfluramine for a period of six months or longer experienced episode/s of pulmonary hypertension" (Dexfenfluramine Side Effects, n.d.). It has side effects on many more parts of your body such as on the endocrine system, on the hepatic system, on the metabolic system, on the nervous system, on the respiratory system, and much more.

Sibutramine

Another drug was removed from the U.S. market in October 2010. But if you're using this medication, you should be aware of the side effects it can have on you in certain cases. For instance, if you have high blood pressure, or any disease that affects your liver or kidneys, suffer from seizures, or fit under the right age category—which should be older than 16 and younger than 65. However, it's always better if you consult a medical professional about which medicine you should take and how much.

Semaglutide (Wegovy or Ozempic)

These two drugs were manufactured because of the drawbacks that liraglutide had. One of the first drugs to be available in both injection and tablet form. Health insurance more often covers Ozempic for diabetic patients, and whether it's included depends on the health insurance. The side effects of this drug are minimal, and in a study, less than five percent of participants suffered from side effects. Those side effects came in the form of stomach problems that did show a significant decrease by the end of the study period (M.D., 2021).

Surgery

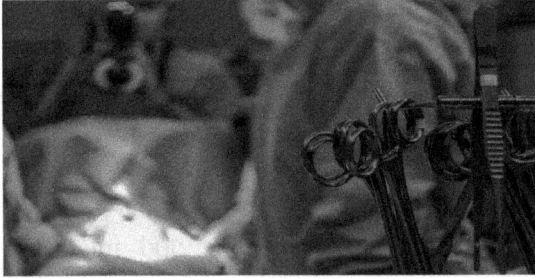

The last treatment methods we will discuss are the surgeries you can opt for to lose weight and become healthier. Let us look at the surgeries that are offered to treat obesity.

Liposuction

The method of the surgery is in its name, where the fat in certain parts of your body is removed through this suction method. In places like your stomach, thighs, and buttocks, fat can be removed through this process. However, this process does not help you with much weight loss like diets and exercise do. This surgery can be done when you have fat stored in a certain part of your body and no amount of exercise or dieting is helping reduce the fat content there. Then, you can consider this surgery as an option to reduce the fat amounts while still maintaining a healthy lifestyle through choices of diet and physical activity. When you get this surgery done, and lose the fat places, it's not guaranteed that the fat won't come back. That's why it's critical to maintain a healthy lifestyle afterwards to prevent fat from reaccumulating in those areas where fat doesn't burn easily.

Just like with any surgery, this one comes with its own risks. You may notice bumpy or itchy skin in the area where the surgery was performed; you may notice fluid has accumulated that needs to be removed with a needle; you may feel numb in that area for a while; your chances of developing organ failure, such as kidney failure, increase; and you may be exposed to any internal punctures, or fat deposits becoming stuck in your blood vessels (Mayo Clinic, 2019).

Gastric Band Surgery

Gastric band surgery happens to decrease your food intake by placing a band around your stomach making it smaller. This makes you full by eating a smaller amount of food, preventing overeating. The band placed on your stomach can be adjusted by adding saline or removing it. It's an effective and proven method of weight loss by the Food and Drug Administration (FDA). The surgery takes up to 60 minutes at most, but the patient will have to prepare the day before and after the surgery. They may also need to take a week off from their day-to-day activities.

Your diet after this surgery will need to change. For the first four weeks, the patient will be strictly on a liquid diet before they can move to softer foods. It can take up to six weeks before the patient can go back to their normal diet with various kinds of food.

The risks of this surgery are as follows. Some people may find themselves rejecting the anesthesia, making the surgical performance difficult. The weight loss from this surgery won't be immediate, and you will still require proper amounts of exercise to start the weight loss as this surgery will just curb your appetite by decreasing your stomach capacity; along with the possibility of the surgery going wrong, and additional procedures being required. However, this surgery is quite beneficial. It's proven to be a long-term weight loss solution—which is not the case with many other surgeries.

Bariatric Surgery

There are two types of surgery that fall under this category and are known specifically as "weight-loss surgeries."

Gastric Bypass

Roux-en-Y (pronounced roo-en-wy) gastric bypass (RYBG) reduces the size of your stomach by decreasing the amount of nutrients absorbed and decreasing your appetite. However, it's the most difficult and time-consuming surgery to perform. There are three alterations that are made during this surgery, and they are stapling the stomach, dividing the small intestine, and relocating the upper small intestine (National Institute of Diabetes, Digestive, and Kidney Diseases, 2019a).

Sleeve Gastrectomy

Vertical sleeve gastrectomy (VSG) is another common surgery performed to reduce weight problems. It again reduces your stomach size and reduces the amount of food you can eat at once, curbing any chances of overeating. It reduces the internal production of hormones that control your hunger needs. Unlike the gastric band surgery method, VSG is permanent as a portion of your stomach is removed and not just restricted.

Both these surgeries can be expensive to perform, and you need to qualify to be able to get them done. You need to have a BMI of 35 or higher, and if no other methods have shown any improvements, you will be able to qualify. The short-term risks for both are blood clots, infections, and diarrhea. And the long-term effects can include hernias, scar tissue, hypoglycemia, etc. While you may not see all these side effects, it's important that you know them, so in case of an emergency, you can act accordingly.

Chapter 11:

Resolving Basic Problems Linked With Obesity

Since there are many problems associated with obesity, you need to be aware of how to tackle them individually as well as when to ask for medical assistance. But there are basic problems that are in your hands to control. For any problem that you find yourself facing, there are certain steps and precautions that you can take without seeking help from medical authorities or drugs. If you know what the problem is, and why it's happening, you can treat it from the start avoiding the severe problems that occur mostly due to ignorance of said problems.

In this chapter, we will talk about the basic problems that can be avoided with a little help from the beginning. Let us look at the problems and what we can do to avoid them becoming disastrous for ourselves.

High Cholesterol

Here are some things you can do to avoid high cholesterol and prevent it from getting worse.

Reduce Intake of Fats

As we're already aware, fat that doesn't get burned into energy gets stored in our body and can have many negative impacts. One of them is becoming bad cholesterol that can then lead to blockages in our arteries and veins leading to multiple heart problems. When you're obese, you know that there's already fat deposits in your body, more than should be. This should make you even more careful when consuming fats because of the bad cholesterol. When you avoid fats in your diet, like red meat and dairy products that are full fat, you can also help reduce the bad cholesterol in your body that causes multiple issues as discussed in the previous chapters.

Quit Smoking

Smoking is a very bad habit generally, but when combined with obesity and high cholesterol, the effects on your body are ten times worse than for a healthy-weight person. When you quit smoking, you will immediately see a positive impact on your cholesterol levels. You will see that not only do the bad cholesterol levels drop, but the good cholesterol levels rise. When you stop smoking, you will see that your blood pressure and heart rate will immediately recover within 20 minutes; within months, your blood circulation will improve; and within a year, your risk of heart problems decreases by 50% (Mayo Clinic, 2018). Therefore, it's extremely important to stop smoking if you want your cholesterol levels to decrease, especially if you have obesity too.

Reduce Alcohol

Alcohol has many negative effects, and when combined with obesity, they make the effects severe. However, a moderate amount of alcohol increases good cholesterol. But this isn't applicable to those who don't drink any alcohol. It's obviously better than any other way, but if you're consuming alcohol, it's important to remember the normal and allowed intake of it. For instance, for a healthy adult, it would be one drink a day. On the other hand, if you have obesity, it's advisable to steer clear of alcohol completely as the many cons outweigh the very few pros. An addiction to alcohol can be the cause and consequence of obesity as discussed in previous chapters, and one should be extremely careful of their alcohol consumption.

Healthier Diet

Consume foods high in omega-3 fatty acids. Bad cholesterol has no effect on omega-3 fatty acids. They do, however, have several other heart-healthy benefits such as lowering blood pressure. Salmon, marlin, sardines, walnuts, and flaxseed are all high in omega-3 fatty acids.

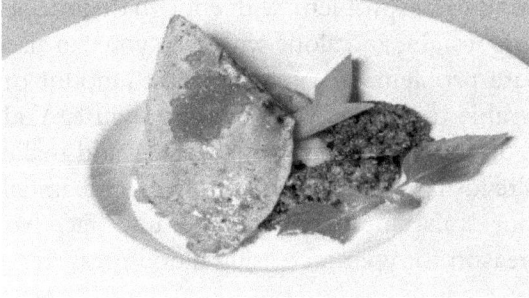

Increase your soluble fiber intake as well. Soluble fiber can help to reduce cholesterol absorption in the bloodstream. Brussels sprouts, kidney beans, oatmeal, apples, and pears contain soluble fiber. Finally, add the whey protein. Many of the benefits attributed to dairy may be credited to whey protein. Whey protein taken as a supplement has been shown in studies to lower bad cholesterol, total cholesterol, and blood pressure (Mayo Clinic, 2018).

High Blood Pressure

High blood pressure can lead to many more issues, so it's important to know how to keep it under control at home and without any medications—in case of emergencies. Here are some practices that can keep your blood pressure in check.

Lose the Excess Weight

The greater your weight, the worse your blood pressure will be. While this is not an immediate solution to the problem, with enough dedication you can tackle obesity by losing weight, and along with that, you can also help your high blood pressure problem. With the smallest amount of weight you lose, you will be able to change your blood pressure. You must keep in mind to be regular in monitoring your weight, and make sure that if you're obese, you're losing weight. As mentioned in the initial chapters, keep track of your waist measurements because fat that accumulates there is a great reason for your increasing blood pressure.

Exercise Regularly

Exercising not only burns fat but also helps lower blood pressure. It doesn't mean just going for a run but doing proper body exercise, so it helps your blood pressure. Since losing weight is also a part of fighting your obesity, it's important to pick an exercise routine that will not only ensure your blood pressure is at a normal rate, but also help you burn fat and lose weight. The better your health, the less concerned you should be about your blood pressure rising again and again; however, it's always better to be sure and keep moving.

Decrease Salt Intake

Sodium in your diet should generally be reduced if you have high blood pressure, especially salt. Even cutting out the smallest quantities of salt can help your blood pressure reduce significantly and almost immediately. According to the Mayo Clinic (2022), "limit sodium to 2,300 mg or less per day. However, a lower sodium intake—1,500 mg a day or less—is ideal for most adults." They also emphasize that sodium, or salt, should not be eliminated completely from the diet, which can lower your blood pressure much more than normal. The best way to reduce salt intake is to eat out less and cook more at home whenever possible. That way you're in control of your salt intake and can adjust accordingly. If you were to eat out, ask for less salt to be added, and check any processed food you buy for its sodium value.

Eat Healthy Food

Eating healthy and being in good shape will automatically lower your blood pressure as a short-term and long-term solution. The healthier you eat, the more you will see that your blood pressure will be at a normal rate. It won't become a habit at once, especially if you have unhealthy eating habits, but starting somewhere can take you a long way. Give yourself one meal per week to have what you like, and with time, make the cheat days farther apart. Do this until eating healthy becomes a daily routine and cheat meals come only occasionally. Eating healthy can also be fun and delicious if you give it a try and the right amount of dedication. You can find delicious alternatives to make you feel as though you aren't missing out on anything.

Heart Attacks and Strokes

Heart attacks can be deadly and painful, and if you find yourself lucky enough to survive one, then it's important to make lifestyle changes that will prevent future heart attacks or strokes. Here are some changes you can make to your daily routine to prevent them.

Manage Your Diabetes

Obesity and diabetes increase your chances of dying from heart disease by 68% and stroke by 16% (American Heart Association, 2015). These numbers are proof that you need to take extra care of your heart so your chances of a heart attack or stroke decrease. When you manage your diabetes by curbing the intake of sugar, you will be able to significantly decrease the risks of heart attacks and strokes. If you're obese with type-1 diabetes inherited, then you will have to take the appropriate medicines along with watching your sugar.

Switch to an Active Lifestyle

The American Heart Association conducted a study where they found promising results regarding exercise helping to reduce heart attacks in participants and now recommend that obese people exercise for prevention. Almost 39% of obese participants were more likely to have heart damage from no regular exercise (n.d.). This is an important way to avoid heart attacks and strokes. However, it's important that you maintain a regular exercise routine and not just once or twice a week. It's the lack of regular exercise that increases your odds of suffering from a heart attack or stroke that could potentially kill you. It has already been discussed how obesity can make your heart condition worse, so now it's time to act upon its prevention before it kills you.

Track Your Meals

Unhealthy meals and overeating can also increase your chances of a heart attack. That's why it's important to track your meals to help prevent heart attacks and strokes. Eating meals heavy in oil and fat can make your risk of heart attack twice as bad if you're already obese. Dr. Aashish Aggarwal, Head of Cardiology at Aakash Healthcare Super Specialty Hospital in New Delhi, spoke about how heavy meals can act as a trigger for a heart attack, and what can be done to reduce the risk of overeating while also adopting a heart-healthy diet (Phelamei, 2020). In summary, you need to spread your food-calorie intake evenly throughout the day and not give in to the temptation of frequent snacks. Moreover, you should avoid oily and fatty foods whenever possible because they're bad for your heart and can increase your chances. Lastly, create a chart that you think will work best for you, filled with healthier options, and stick to that plan strictly. The more room you leave for excuses, the harder it will be for you to prevent the worst effects of heart attacks and strokes on yourself.

Maintain Healthy Weight

The American Heart Association (n.d.) conducted a study with women, where they reached the conclusion that losing even 10% of their body weight reduced heart-attack risk. This proved that maintaining a healthy weight after losing weight is also important in reducing the risk of heart attacks and strokes. You can maintain a healthy weight by being aware of what the ideal weight range is, where you're at in that range, and what you can do that will help you lose weight quickly and in a healthy way. Once you beat your obesity, and get back to the ideal weight range, it's important to remember that weight is not a permanent change. If you forget to keep track and be careful, then you will start to gain weight again and will be faced with the risks of heart attacks and strokes all over.

Keep Track of Your Blood Pressure and Cholesterol

As these are the factors that add to the risks of suffering a heart attack or stroke, it's important to keep maintaining them as well. If they get out of hand, then you will have to take the necessary measures to get them back to the normal range. If you don't know about your blood pressure and cholesterol, when it rises or drops, leading to a possible heart attack or stroke, you won't know the exact cause of it. As the saying goes, it's better to be safe than sorry.

Low Self-Esteem and Confidence

Another problem arising from obesity is our confidence in ourselves that can also be helped without the use of drugs, and here's how.

Counsel Yourself Toward Positivity

Open your mind to possibilities that lie above all the social challenges you may face when dealing with obesity. There will always be people who won't understand your mental health space and how much you might be struggling to fight obesity. But don't stop just because of them. Find people who are positive in nature, and if there are none, then you become your own motivator. Don't forget that at this day and age, you can seek help professionally as well to help your confidence. Once you focus and work on yourself, becoming more motivated to fight obesity, you will be able to glide through life without being self-conscious and lacking confidence in yourself.

Motivate Yourself to Lose Weight

Low self-esteem can also make you lose hope of ever losing weight and being physically attractive to anyone; however, you can use that as a motivator and fight obesity even harder to achieve your desired weight and regain your confidence. Being confident is loving yourself, and you need to love yourself to be healthy; although it's not a prerequisite, with obesity being a disease you can control, you can easily use it as a motivation to get your confidence back. One way to do that is by looking into the mirror and saying, "I am not my weight, and I will love myself regardless."

Meditate

Meditation can be a great way to let go of all the negativity around you and learn to love yourself by building a stronger connection. Sometimes, we tend to reciprocate negativity by either responding in anger or accepting it and lashing out at ourselves. What that does in return is make us hate ourselves, and instead of fighting obesity, you might just give in and make things worse for yourself. So, meditation can separate you from the hateful comments, and find a positive bond with yourself, making you motivated to lose weight and become healthy as well. Aside from the goal that you will regain your confidence, meditation will help you in all other aspects of your life too.

Inactive Lifestyle

If you struggle with working out and following a set routine for more than a day, then here are some ways you can start to become active more frequently.

Start Simple

When starting off with the goal of losing weight, and becoming more active for your overall health, it's not advisable to jump right into an extensive routine. However serious your problem may seem, if you jump into the extensive routines, you will find them too strenuous and off-putting at the time, resulting in giving up. That's why it's important that you start slow and give yourself some slack at the beginning. Then as you move forward, you can always get into it more. Some ways you can try to be active are:

- Ride a bicycle to work or university.
- Walk if it's under a five-mile radius.
- At night, or when it's pleasant out, visit the nearest park, and take a lap around it.
- If you like a certain sport, play it with your friends, or practice it alone.
- When you have free time, don't resort to electronics; go outside for a walk.
- Make your workouts simple and fun by bringing along a friend or your spouse.

Frequent Walking and Jogging

Like mentioned above, take any free time you get and turn it into a walk or jog. It doesn't have to be boring. You can try many ways to make it seem simple and not like a task that you must do. For instance, when you decide to go for a walk, you can phone a friend that you have lost touch with and catch up with them during your walk. You can bring along someone and talk to them during the walk to make it seem like fun for you and not a chore. You can also listen to music while jogging or walking and have some time to get your thoughts aligned and focused again. You don't even have to remove time. You can just simply choose to walk to places you have to work at between meetings, or take the stairs instead of the elevator, and if time isn't an issue, you can always take the long way around places within your office. Just get yourself moving, and you will find yourself slowly becoming active.

Don't Sit For Too Long

Begin to develop the habit of staying active on a regular basis. If you work a desk job, then it's a good idea to keep constant timers that would remind you to get up, stretch, and have a small walk, even if it's just around the office. If you're constantly moving from one place to another, for instance, for meetings, then it would be better if you walk wherever you can or keep it outdoors if possible. The fresh air can also help to get you active. Sometimes, sitting at a desk all day can make us tired with minimal activity from our side. That's why it's also better that whenever you take breaks, you get out of the office and head somewhere where there's fresh air to rejuvenate you and give you some energy to get active even in your workplace.

Depression

As discussed in the previous chapters, depression can be the outcome of obesity too, and while you can always reach out and seek help, here are some ways you can help yourself with depression.

Engage in Productive Activities

When in depression, you might find it hard to get out of bed, and that can delay your course of fighting obesity. It can hinder your motivation and can also reverse any progress you have made. So, when you feel the depression kicking in, it's a good idea to push yourself to be productive. It doesn't have to be a major goal in your life. But getting out of bed to have a healthy meal and go for a jog in nature can be a start. Even the simplest of activities you push yourself to do will help you in the long run to fight obesity. Find joy in the simplest of activities that you do even if life generally makes you sad. If you get out of bed on time, be happy about it. If you chose a healthy meal over takeout, be happy about the choice you made—even if it doesn't make much of a difference.

Meditate Regularly

Just like with self-esteem, meditating can help you come out of depression. When you meditate, you not only practice your breathing but also focus on yourself. Your body and your emotions too. When you give your emotions free space to feel, they won't get bottled up, and you won't feel overwhelmed by them. You will also give yourself the space and time to heal and sharpen your focus on your goals. That's why it's important that you bring meditation into your life to help with your depression.

Chapter 12

Methods to Keep Your Life on a Weight-Loss Track

You might find it difficult to track how much weight you need to lose, and how far along you are in finding quick and effective methods you can introduce into your life that can help you on your weight-loss journey. This chapter will help you track your weight loss, and provide some tips on the do's and don'ts when fighting obesity. We will cover topics like making a diet chart; drinking lots of water; exercising regularly; the effects of stress; and so much more.

Download a Daily Meal Tracker

There are many meal trackers available, free of charge, that can help you track the calories you consume with whatever you ingest. You can add the item and the portion size for it to calculate the calorie count, and it will subtract it from your daily count, so you don't have to remember everything at once. These meal trackers may not give you the exact count, but it's more accurate than calculating the calories by yourself. Furthermore, by entering your weight and height into the app, they will calculate your BMI and the amount of weight you need to lose. Some apps will also provide you with a plan to follow, but you may have to purchase it.

Make a Diet Chart

A diet chart can be made by you, or a nutritionist, or can be found online as well. Diet charts help you in two main ways: to count your calories and to save money on expensive foods. Your diet chart will consist of foods that you can and cannot eat throughout the day. This can include some items you can eat at certain times of the day to help you get more energy and avoid them towards the end of the day. Moreover, there will be certain food groups that you might have to limit and certain food groups that you need to have more of. You may also be asked to avoid certain items that may add more weight than they help you gain energy from. For instance, fruits, like mangoes and bananas, and vegetables, like beetroot and spinach, should be avoided.

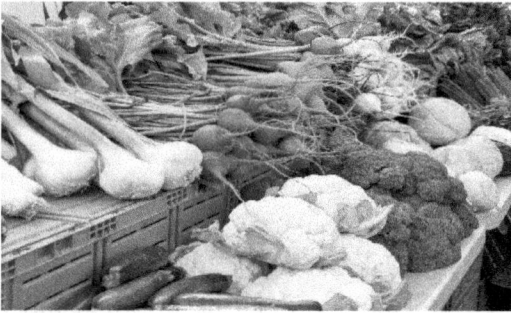

Eat Small, Regular Meals

Eating small but regular meals can help you track and control your weight loss. This isn't about eating at regular intervals, but about eating at the right times and in the right amounts. Some people resort to skipping meals to lose weight, and that just results in them getting tired very easily and engaging in more snacking habits. Instead of that, it's recommended that you eat a proper meal during the appropriate times—without overeating—and don't resort to snacking very often. In fact, with the goal of losing weight, snacking should be completely left behind.

Eat a Balanced Diet

Having a balanced diet is a very important aspect in people's lives, and most importantly for obese people. This is because we often forget the food pyramid and how much of each food group should be consumed which lets the fat build up in our bodies, resulting in obesity. An obese person should keep in mind that the food groups should be consumed in the proper amounts. For instance, consuming fat and sugar during the day should be controlled and less than when compared with fruits, vegetables, and proteins. Your diet should be rich in fiber and proteins and low in fats and refined carbs. As an alternative to refined carbs, you can opt for refined grains as they contain all the healthy aspects of refined carbs. Moreover, indulging in seafood is better than choosing red meat as an obese person as it can increase protein levels without eating a high quantity of it. In this example, you can opt for chicken or fish like salmon. Furthermore, the best option for losing weight when obese is to increase fruit and vegetable consumption. This doesn't mean stop eating other types of food, but carving out the fat can always help, just as increasing the intake of fruits and vegetables does. Lastly, it's important that your sugar level is kept to a minimum. Even for a healthy person, the sugar intake should be less, and for obese people, that needs to be taken care of more carefully. Your sugar intake as an obese person should be less than 5% of your total calories, and for a healthy person, it's 10% of the total calorie intake (Sengupta, 2018).

Avoid Junk Food

It should be a given that when you start to gain weight, you cut down on fast and junk foods. This is because they're made of ingredients that are unhealthy and easily add fat to your body's storage. However, it's so easily available and advertised to look appealing that you may find it hard to resist eating it. But it's important to know your goal in life is to fight obesity and survive it. This would require you to cut back on junk food whenever possible. If you're at the morbid obesity stage, then this type of food is absolutely forbidden as it does way more harm than benefit.

Plan Your Meals Wisely

Once you know the average calorie count you need to get sufficient energy throughout the day, it's important to plan your meals accordingly, so you don't exceed the calorie count due to ignorance, or a mistake in calculating, resulting in overeating. The meals you need to plan out are breakfast, lunch, an evening snack, and dinner. Each of these should be healthy and provide you with as much energy as you need until the next meal. You should not cut down on calories so much that you resort to frequent snacking. In fact, if you can avoid the evening snack and make it to dinner without feeling too tired and snacking, then it's better. But if you absolutely need to snack, then ensure that it's healthy and won't add to your weight. For example, instead of snacking on a burrito, snack on some dry fruits. Similarly, when planning out your three meals of the day, make sure they're healthy and filled with nutrients rather than fats and sugar that may provide instant energy but will also make you gain weight instead of losing it.

Drink Plenty of Water

Water is the best solution to losing weight and many other problems. Along with keeping you well hydrated, drinking plenty of water throughout the day will also help you lose weight. How that happens is that water helps burn your calories faster. In a study conducted, women who were obese were given 34 oz of water to drink daily, and when checked, the results showed a 4.4-pound weight loss because of water (Stookey et al., 2008). Use this method, combined with other weight-loss plans, and you will see a significant decrease in your weight. Moreover, this is something you don't need to make time to do; you can carry water wherever you go and keep sipping from your bottle.

Exercise Regularly

It's vital that you exercise, and you may notice it being mentioned many times above already. However, exercising is something that can be done by yourself too, and something that has proven to help with losing weight. The amount of exercise you do will increase the weight-loss rate. But the important factor here is to do it regularly. Because if you skip a day or two, you will find it's easier to give yourself slack, and that can result in you skipping out on your exercise more often. Eventually, your activity rate will decrease, and you will start associating yourself with the phrase "couch potato" more often.

Chapter 13:

What You Gain When You Lose Weight

Losing weight can be tough and a hard-working achievement, but when you lose weight, you gain many benefits in life. You no longer must worry about suffering from the endless diseases that could potentially kill you. You can live freely and even start enjoying the various aspects of life that you could not enjoy with obesity looming over your head. You increase your chances of having a successful and happy life. On top of that, the loved ones around you are also benefiting from you losing weight as they no longer must spend their lives worrying about you financially, mentally, and physically. The following are some of the advantages of losing excess weight.

Health Benefits

Losing weight can help prevent and cure type-2 diabetes. According to the American Heart Association (n.d.), losing even five to seven percent of body weight can help prevent type-2 diabetes by 58%. Losing weight can help lower blood glucose levels to an ideal range and let you function through life without worrying much about your sugar levels. However, it's advisable that you keep checking your blood sugar levels whenever possible, even after losing weight. This is because after losing weight some might let go of the control on their dietary restrictions that can then cause a relapse in type-2 diabetes and obesity. After losing weight, you can start to release a little control over your restrictions, but make sure you don't let go completely.

The next health benefit is your blood pressure coming back to normal without any medication needed. Unless you have another disease that can raise your blood pressure, losing weight can lower your blood pressure to normal levels. As mentioned above, you should always keep checking your weight, and your blood pressure, and be informed in case of any emergency. Once you lose weight, however, you will see that your blood pressure will also regulate, and the doctors may also ask you to stop any medications that you used to take specifically for controlling your blood pressure due to obesity. To get your blood pressure levels back to normal, it's highly important that you lose abdominal fat as that's the major reason linked to obesity and high blood pressure levels.

Moreover, as you lose weight, your mobility levels will also improve. With the excess weight of even 10 pounds, it can add up to 40 pounds of pressure on your knees. Which is why losing weight can also make it easier for you to perform tasks without tiring yourself more than usual. A simple trip up the stairs will be easier with better mobility than having excess weight on your body weighing you down. You will also experience fewer instances of joint pain that would happen frequently when you're overweight.

As discussed in the previous chapters, losing weight plays a big part in reducing your chances of suffering from heart attacks and strokes. Furthermore, losing weight reduces the severity of the attacks and their aftereffects. For example, when an obese person suffers a stroke or heart attack, there's a very good possibility of death, and even if they don't die, their mental and physical health deteriorates drastically. But when a normal person suffers from a stroke or heart attack, they have more of a fighting chance to get out of the experience with minimal effects. This is an added benefit to losing weight since you get more of a fighting chance when facing heart attacks and strokes.

Lastly, losing weight has the benefit of preventing various other diseases. By losing weight and fighting obesity, diseases like cancer and sleeping problems can all be reduced and prevented. There's no guarantee that you won't get these diseases, but without obesity snatching away your life, your chances of getting these diseases decrease significantly. Moreover, you won't have to fight off so many disorders at once like blood pressure problems and sleep apnea that often occur when you have obesity.

Lifestyle Benefits

Along with many health benefits as discussed above, there are also lifestyle benefits that will come along with losing weight. Firstly, it will help build your confidence. Once you lose weight, you will find yourself loving and accepting your body better which will make you more confident when approaching people, attending meetings, and tackling any social gathering in your life. Confidence doesn't necessarily depend on your being confident in your physical appearance, but also how you carry yourself and how strong your mental health is. For instance, obesity also causes depression which can also make you lose your confidence. Just like that, losing weight can help with your depression and make you more hopeful about your life which will show improvement in your self-esteem.

Secondly, you can rediscover your old friendships and relationships that you lost touch with for several reasons revolving around obesity. As we have seen above, obesity can take a toll on your relationships for many different reasons that can be resolved with losing weight and fighting obesity. You may have found it hard to keep up with your friends during your obesity and have slowly lost touch with them, but once you lose weight, you can focus on rekindling that spark rather than worrying about your health. Similarly, it works the same way for romantic relationships. You might have been so preoccupied with the problems of obesity that it took away time for you to get out there and meet new people, but now that you don't have to worry as much, you can go out and meet some people and find someone who will keep you dedicated to staying healthy.

Another lifestyle benefit from losing weight is improving your sex life. With obesity looming over head, not only will you find it hard to perform sexually and keep your partner satisfied, but you will also face many issues regarding reproduction. However, once you lose weight, you also reduce any chances of not performing well sexually. It will not become a chore for you, and you will also be able to enjoy the sexual activity that you engage in.

Moreover, you will also find that your stress levels will be lower by losing weight. This is because you will be able to focus on your work and personal life without worrying about obesity and its problems. The financial stress itself will decrease drastically as you will now be making healthier choices that in the long term will help you save on costs and use them somewhere more beneficial. You will have more time to put into your work life also reducing stress from coping at work. Less stress means better health both mentally and physically. Your performance level will shoot up, and you will be able to prioritize tasks according to importance and not necessarily according to what gets you the least tired.

Lastly, losing weight will help you sleep better. It will help with your sleeping patterns in the sense that you will be able to fall asleep much faster and deeper than with obesity. Your sleep apnea will also see drastic improvements, giving you a stable and restful night of sleep without any disturbance because of obesity. It will also make you more comfortable when sleeping. With being overweight, you may have also faced the issue of not being able to be comfortable in your bed and needing assistance with getting in and out of bed that will all go away once you lose weight. Better sleep at night will reduce your daytime tiredness and keep you energetic throughout the day.

Financial Benefits

Your monthly expenses revolving around obesity will drop drastically when you lose weight and fight obesity. Sure, you won't be able to choose the cheaper option in food as they are fast foods and very unhealthy, but with the overall saving on surgeries and treatments, you will be able to save a lot of money for better use. Many medications to treat the problems that arise from obesity are expensive, and since they're long-term, you must invest a lot. And in the unfortunate event of a surgery, it can really take a hit on your savings, and in some cases, even put you in debt.

That brings us to diets that help with losing weight. Even though healthy food is slightly on the expensive scale, and sometimes, to exercise you may need to get a gym membership, or purchase equipment if you work out at home, the total cost of these expenses added up is still less when you add in the risks of surgeries and hospital bills when obesity becomes worse. Think of losing weight as an investment that will help your cash flow in the future from hefty expenses.

Chapter 14

World Health Organization on Obesity

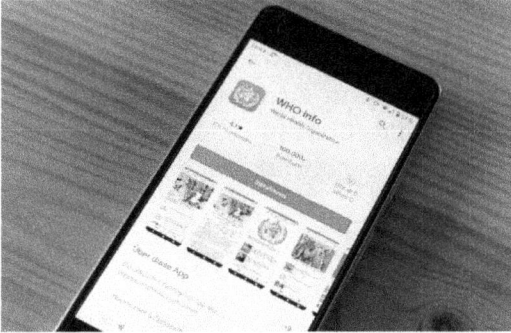

The World Health Organization (WHO), an organization founded by the United Nations in 1948, helps keep the world safe by prioritizing health concerns worldwide. On obesity, the WHO has done extensive research and found out the major causes and impacts of obesity on people. They have done this so they can help identify the problem and help the affected people around the world tackle it. WHO has set out guidelines and initiatives to help stop the problem of obesity and how, in different regions, the causes and treatments must be different.

Obesity—A Global Epidemic

The World Health Organization has declared obesity a global epidemic, or "globesity," because of its rapid spread in almost all regions of the world. Apart from a few countries, obesity is being ignored by most, and as stated by WHO, "if immediate action is not taken, millions will suffer from an array of serious health disorders." They have also identified that obesity is more commonly found in females, while in males, just being overweight is most common. What happened once they announced obesity as an epidemic?

Since 1990, WHO has sent out many guidelines that help spread awareness and provide action plans to help the people who suffer from obesity. For instance, they have sent out publications regarding different tips to follow to help with obesity, one of them being the importance of reducing sodium—salt—in our diets. They have also created multiple resolutions, one of which is to replace trans-fat and fat-free products by 2023. Their publications also focus more on the young who are affected by obesity. This is because childhood obesity affects their whole future, and in general, the future of the world. On top of that, they have a helpline that anyone can call and get in touch with, and they're holding

multiple events to spread awareness and educate people on the negative impacts of obesity.

World Obesity Day

On World Obesity Day in 2022, the World Health Organization highlighted how obesity can make the impacts of Covid-19 even worse. Moreover, they focused on the strategy plan to prevent obesity that lasts over the timeline of 2019–2023. Here are certain aims of their strategy plan:

- tax on sugar
- eliminate subside of fats and oils
- introduce a healthy provision of healthy foods
- make the food nutrition label on products mandatory
- recommendation of food to purchase and what to avoid
- increase physical activity action plan
- conducting campaigns on healthy dieting
- promote more breastfeeding for children

They use this action plan and many more statistical analyses to help spread awareness of how obesity has had a huge impact and how it harms us additionally in the Covid-19 era. It helps us understand that obesity is not a one-time problem that attacks us alone, but rather weakens our ability to fight off new diseases. WHO also records that obesity is spreading in countries where there's also starvation raising a whole lot of controversy that should not happen. In parts of the world where starvation and malnutrition are serious issues, there are also rising cases of obesity. Where food should be saved and given out, people are choosing to overeat and waste food.

Obesity Statistics and Data

Let's look at some statistical data by the World Health Organization on obesity in all age groups.

- Obesity now is three times more than it was in the 1970s.
- Almost 650 million people in 2016 were obese, out of that 40% were women.
- Over 39 million children were obese in 2020—showing the increase of obesity in children.

WHO (2021) published few tips on how to help fight obesity and prevent it from happening again—supporting the content in the previous chapters—and they are:

- limit energy intake from total fats and sugars
- increase consumption of fruit and vegetables as well as legumes, whole grains, and nuts
- engage in regular physical activity (60 minutes a day for children, and 150 minutes spread through the week for adults)

Obesity Prevention Framework by WHO

Their prevention framework is from 2019–2023 as mentioned above. The aims and strategies will be measured by how the countries respond to their call-to-action plan. One way to track that is by ensuring all countries have a sugar tax added that will decrease the amount of sugar products consumed. Next, a country's distribution of healthy foods in schools, universities, hospitals, etc. can help the people adapt to healthy food faster. An additional point would be to make healthy foods affordable and not expensive which can make people deteriorate back to fast foods and unhealthy options. Furthermore, prevention of marketing of unhealthy foods should also be restricted in countries where such food marketing is the major cause of obesity. WHO mentions, "Mandatory restrictions to eliminate all forms of marketing of foods high in fat, sugar, and salt to children and adolescents (up to age 18) are in place across all media" (2019).

Chapter 15:

Trending Misconceptions About Weight Loss

Just like with many other disorders, obesity has many misconceptions that can lead to people being unaware of or believing in certain myths that can make the disorder worse. Learning about the right causes and impacts of obesity can also help when fighting obesity or helping someone struggling with it. Some of the common misconceptions are not knowing which foods make you gain weight and which of these foods are truly healthy but get put off because of the misconception of gaining weight, or assuming that all healthy foods are expensive. In this chapter, we will be confronting some of these misconceptions about obesity and helping to clear them.

Obesity Is Not a Diseased Condition

A major misconception about obesity is that people think it's not a disease but a choice, and this is incorrect. As discussed above, obesity is caused by a variety of factors and is not just caused by overeating. That's why people cannot generalize that obesity isn't a disease. Even if done by the choice of overeating, and eating unhealthy foods only, it's still a disease. Merriam-Webster defines disease as "a condition of the living animal or plant body or of one of its parts that impairs normal functioning and is typically manifested by distinguishing signs and symptoms" (n.d.). This definition shows us that obesity is also a disease as it affects one or many parts of your body and keeps them from functioning normally. Like any other disease, obesity also has its own signs and symptoms to distinguish it.

Once people start to realize that obesity is a disease, spreading awareness and educating people on the impacts of obesity will become easier. It also becomes hard to ignore obesity when the seriousness of this disease is well known. Take cancer as an example: when someone we know, or if we are diagnosed with it, we don't treat it lightly and act upon it fast because our lives are on the line; similarly, when someone we know or ourselves are diagnosed with obesity, we should treat it much like cancer in the sense that our lives are on the line.

Carbs Can Make You Gain Weight

Carbs themselves don't make you gain weight. It's the excessive amount that leads people to easily believe that carbs make you gain weight. The same goes for fat. If you recall the food pyramid, fats are a part of it and are not omitted from it. This proves that fat should, in fact, be a part of your meals, but in a moderate portion. However small the portion may be, you need to consume fat and carbs in your diet. Carbs, in specific, can be both good and bad depending on the way they're consumed. For example, the carbs that are present in a chocolate cupcake are also present in a banana. But eating a cupcake will make you think you're gaining weight, and eating a banana seems healthy. This example is a great way to show that it's the quantity and the type of food that's consumed that matter. The banana will give you more energy during the day than the cupcake will.

Healthy Food Is Expensive

The notion that healthy food is expensive is vast and generalized. It puts people under the notion that opting for any healthy food is going to be expensive. That's not the case. When you opt to make a meal at home, using healthy and fresh ingredients, it will be significantly cheaper than dining out. Making a meal from scraps can even turn out to be cheaper than takeout in many circumstances. That's why the notion that healthy food is expensive is a misconception. However, organic food is expensive. But not all healthy food is organic, and not all organic food is healthy. It's just a matter of knowing which foods are healthier among the advertised and expensive products.

Another reason why healthy food may seem expensive to any person nowadays is because of the minimal advertising of those foods, and the increased advertising of fast food and dining out. Because of the restaurant industry's advertising that captures the attention of the people and the lack of advertising on eating at home (as any market doesn't profit much from it), the people are led to believe that healthy food is expensive, and usually opt for the easier and cheaper alternative of fast food.

Exercise Is the Only Solution to Lose Weight

Although exercise is one option to lose weight, it's not the only one. You can also diet and make other lifestyle choices that can help you lose weight drastically. On top of that, you can also use medical help in the form of drugs or surgery to treat obesity and lose weight. So, while exercise is an effective option to lose weight, it's a misconception to think it's the only choice. Sometimes, exercise alone may not be enough to help you lose weight. You will need to add other options with it to consistently lose weight.

Furthermore, exercise doesn't always have to be hardcore and push you to extreme limits. It can also be going out for a run and getting more physical in your activities. You can swim, cycle, or hike, and it will still be counted as exercise.

Slimming Pills Are Safe

Assuming or thinking that slimming pills are safe is a dangerous misconception. It may be an easy option to lose weight, but the impact it can have on your body can be permanent and irreversible. While obesity is reversible, and you can use other methods—that will require more dedication and hard work—that will also help you lose weight and fight obesity, It's important that your slimming pills are prescribed, and that you know the possible side effects of them in case of any emergencies. Taking slimming pills that aren't prescribed can be extremely dangerous and can possibly have side effects that affect your life worse than obesity and can also possibly lead to heart failure.

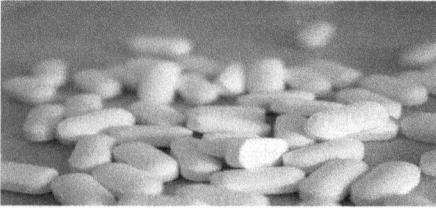

Starving Burns Extra Calories

Skipping out on meals will not only *not* help you lose weight any faster but will also make you weaker. Losing weight doesn't mean that you skip out on eating but means to eat the correct amounts of nutrients that are needed throughout the day. When you start to skip meals, thinking that you will lose weight faster by doing so, you will also lose out on your needed energy and find yourself getting tired very easily. This can affect your productivity at your place of work or study. Moreover, if you skip meals, your hunger will eventually reach a point where you will resort to snacking. Snacking is unhealthy because you're not waiting at the proper times, and you eat more than needed because of the immense hunger. Firstly, if you eat at the wrong time, your whole eating schedule will get messed up. For example, you will snack in the evening from dying hunger then have a late dinner of which most nutrients won't be needed as you will soon head to bed. That's why eating meals properly and at the correct time is very important.

Chapter   16:
Inspiration   for   Weight-Loss
Transformation

In the current situation, obesity is not entirely ignored by the people. There are a good number of people in all parts of the world who are battling obesity and many who are spreading awareness and educating people all around the world. This is one step closer in battling obesity. Once people know the problem, they can find out and work towards the solution. Many famous people have also battled or are battling obesity which gives us an inspiration to do the same for ourselves and the people we love who get diagnosed with obesity. Let us look at some examples of famous celebrities that have battled obesity.

Tom Arnold—American Actor and Comedian

The infamous actor and comedian Tom Arnold explained his story for People.com. He narrated how he set a goal to lose weight, and what tactics he used to achieve the weight loss. His success was pushed because of the birth of his child and the undying support from his wife. Moreover, he said that his success also came from discipline and following the routine. Another key factor in his success was that he never gave up pushing himself even when his schedule used to change. He didn't use working out as an excuse to not help with the baby; in fact, he said, "If I'm on baby duty, and I'm watching the monitor in the gym, and he starts crying, I write down my 16 minutes or whatever and come back later to finish." With a career and other duties, if a celebrity can do it, so can we! Additionally, he did eat properly and didn't starve himself, thinking it would help him lose more weight; he says that he used to eat four meals per day but in smaller quantities, so it gave him the right amount of energy required for him to perform his tasks (Lewis, 2020).

Pete Alonso—American Baseball Player

An athlete with an obesity history is the perfect motivation for the sports lovers among us. Pete Alonso overcame his obesity and became a major league baseball player (MLB) and reached the position of the second-fastest player. This is a motivational story because this shows us that obesity doesn't limit us from our dreams and goals if we choose to fight it. Obesity being a reversible disease can give every one of us the chance to overcome our battles and achieve the life we deserve. Peter told ESPN that he was bullied as a child for being obese, and he turned those insults into motivation and worked hard to become healthy again (Thompson, 2021).

Caleb Swanigan—American Basketball Player

Another athlete that had obesity in his history. Caleb Swanigan had many environmental factors and genetics that led him to obesity. He grew up in a household that would choose unhealthy foods over healthy food because it was cheaper. They used to indulge in whatever they could get as food was also sometimes a scarcity. When that happened, and Caleb would eat whatever he could, he gained weight drastically. In eighth grade, it's believed that he weighed 400 pounds. However, for his case, his passion for basketball got him motivated. Caleb was even good at this as his brother quoted that, "He had the moves, but he just couldn't move" (Thompson, 2021). It was in his luck when his brother got an NFL player to agree to adopt him and raise him to help with obesity. The American basketball player's life changed from that moment. He began exercising hard under the guidance of the NFL player and reduced his weight. Sometimes, we need the support and guidance of our loved ones or role models—wherever possible—to get back in good shape and achieve our dreams.

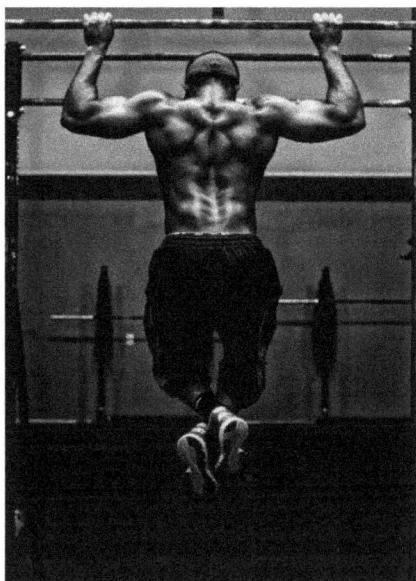

Jessica Simpson—American Singer and Actress

Just like many other women, Jessica Simpson gained weight from her pregnancy. However, she battled obesity after birth not just one time but three. Inspiration from this singer and actress can encourage many women who need to find the right motivation to get back in shape after pregnancy. She achieved this three times by lifestyle changes and a lot of dedication.

Jessica Simpson said for *Today* (Newcomb & Steinhilber, 2020):

> "I call it determined patience. I believe in setting small goals for yourself because in my life and how I've done it, there's easy ways to throw in the towel and just feel like it's impossible. So, the small goals for me are what helped me achieve the main goal."

Conclusion

This is it. Your knowledge on obesity, its causes, and impacts, is complete. In this book, we talked about various topics. Here's a short summary for what was in the chapters. Each number coincides with its chapter in the book.

1. Starting with obesity in the childhood years, this chapter covers the reasons, medical issues, social challenges, and helping tips for childhood obesity.
2. Learning the different choices that result in obesity is covered in this chapter. From lifestyle choices to health-related issues to genetic issues. It's deeply covered in this chapter.
3. Moving onto the different categories of obesity. Which were android and gynoid obesity. Your BMI also defines what condition you have. Whether you're underweight, overweight, or obese.
4. Then talking about the diagnosis to know whether you or someone you love has obesity. You can find out from self-screening or by conducting certain lab tests.
5. This chapter highlights the risks of heart attacks and strokes that obesity has on your body with an additional section on what substances boost that risk.
6. This chapter covers other health issues that are associated with obesity from cancer to acanthosis nigricans.
7. Then moving on to the social challenges that you might face with obesity. This includes being bullied, low quality of living, missing out on opportunities, bad relationships with people, and finding difficulty while traveling.
8. Talking about the psychological trauma that revolves around obesity is very important and is covered in this chapter. Like

getting hit with depression, stress, and anxiety, having low self-confidence, and hating yourself.

9. The financial cost revolving around obesity is also an important area to cover as people need to know how obesity will empty your bank accounts from surgeries to difficulty to get the right things in life; obese people must spend a lot.

10. Moving on to the different treatments for obesity. This chapter talks about different therapies and surgical options.

11. This chapter helps you resolve some of the basic problems you might face with effective solutions. Some are instant results while some will give you results from consistency.

12. This chapter helps you keep track of your weight loss. It shows you different ways of how you can keep track of your weight loss, and how to keep up the consistency when losing weight.

13. In this chapter, we covered some of the benefits you will get when you lose weight. This can also serve as a motivational chapter to get you to lose the excess weight.

14. Then talking about what the World Health Organization has to say on obesity, and what they have done to spread awareness and help prevent it.

15. We tackled all the myths and misconceptions revolving around obesity in this chapter.

16. Lastly, giving you some inspirational stories of famous people to get you motivated to lose weight and fight obesity.

Now it's time to get started fighting obesity and help your loved ones fight it too. In this advancing world, it's important to not turn a blind eye to obesity. If this book helped you in even the tiniest way, leave a review behind to help us and help others who are struggling with obesity as well!

References

Ali, Y. (2016, December 29). *The Many Different Types of Obesity*. Verywell Health. https://www.verywellhealth.com/different-types-of-obesity-4121042

Amiri, M., & Ramezani Tehrani, F. (2020). *Potential Adverse Effects of Female and Male Obesity on Fertility: A Narrative Review*. International Journal of Endocrinology and Metabolism, 18(3). https://doi.org/10.5812/ijem.101776

Anorexia. (2014, December 19). Harvard Health. https://www.health.harvard.edu/diseases-and-conditions/anorexia

Baffi, C. W., Winnica, D. E., & Holguin, F. (2015). *Asthma and Obesity: Mechanisms and Clinical Implications*. Asthma Research and Practice, 1(1). https://doi.org/10.1186/s40733-015-0001-7

Bakalar, N. (2009, June 8). *Childhood: Obesity Linked to Sleep Disorder*. The New York Times. https://www.nytimes.com/2009/06/09/health/research/09chil.html

Bjarnadottir, A. (2017, June 4). *How Drinking More Water Can Help You Lose Weight*. Healthline. https://www.healthline.com/nutrition/drinking-water-helps-with-weight-loss

Boh, P. (2021, March 3). *Obesity and Alzheimer's Disease—Risk?* ReaDementia. https://readementia.com/obesity-and-alzheimers-disease

Can Lifestyle Changes Benefit Your Cholesterol? (2018). Mayo Clinic. https://www.mayoclinic.org/diseases-conditions/high-blood-cholesterol/in-depth/reduce-cholesterol/art-20045935

Can Triglycerides Affect My Heart Health? (n.d.). Mayo Clinic. https://www.mayoclinic.org/diseases-conditions/high-blood-cholesterol/in-depth/triglycerides/art-20048186

Cardiovascular Diseases (CVDs). (2021, June 11). World Health Organization. https://www.who.int/news-room/fact-sheets/detail/cardiovascular-diseases-(cvds)

Causes and Consequences of Childhood Obesity. (2022, March 21). Centers for Disease Control and Prevention. https://www.cdc.gov/obesity/basics/causes.html

Chatterjee, S. (2022, September 9). *10 Types Of Acanthosis Nigricans (Velvety Skin) & Ayurvedic* Cure. Vedix. https://vedix.com/blogs/articles/acanthosis-nigricans-treatment

Cherney, K. (2022, July 28). *Everything You've Ever Wanted to Know About Bariatric Surgery.* Healthline. https://www.healthline.com/health/obesity/bariatric-surgery#risks

Christiansen, S. (2019, July 27). *How Obesity Is Diagnosed.* Verywell Health. https://www.verywellhealth.com/how-obesity-is-diagnosed-4690037

Colino, S. (n.d.). *Obesity and Heart Disease: What's the Connection?* Everyday Health. https://www.everydayhealth.com/heart-disease/obesity-heart-disease-whats-connection

Controlling the Global Obesity Epidemic. (2020). World Health Organization. https://www.who.int/activities/controlling-the-global-obesity-epidemic

Corica, D., Aversa, T., Valenzise, M., Messina, M. F., Alibrandi, A., De Luca, F., & Wasniewska, M. (2018). *Does Family History of Obesity, Cardiovascular, and Metabolic Diseases Influence Onset and Severity of Childhood Obesity?* Frontiers in Endocrinology, 9. https://doi.org/10.3389/fendo.2018.00187

Crönlein, T. (2016). *Insomnia and Obesity.* Current Opinion in Psychiatry, 29(6), 409–412. https://doi.org/10.1097/yco.0000000000000284

Dare, S., Mackay, D. F., & Pell, J. P. (2015). *Relationship Between Smoking and Obesity: A Cross-Sectional Study of 499,504 Middle-Aged Adults in the UK General Population.* PLOS ONE, 10(4). https://doi.org/10.1371/journal.pone.0123579

Davidson, K. (2021, November 30). *How Many Calories Do I Burn in a Day?* Healthline. https://www.healthline.com/health/fitness-exercise/how-many-calories-do-i-burn-a-day

Definition & Facts for Bariatric Surgery. (2019, November 10). National Institute of Diabetes and Digestive and Kidney Diseases. https://www.niddk.nih.gov/health-information/weight-management/bariatric-surgery/definition-facts

Diabetes and Your Heart. (2020, January 31). Centers for Disease Control and Prevention. https://www.cdc.gov/diabetes/library/features/diabetes-and-heart.html

Doheny, K. (2009, August 22). *Childhood Obesity Can Lead to Heart Disease.* WebMD.

https://www.webmd.com/children/features/children-and-heart-disease-whats-wrong-with-this-picture

Durbin, K. (n.d.). *Orlistat: Uses, Dosage, & Side Effects*. Drugs.com. https://www.drugs.com/orlistat.html

Exercise Minimizes Heart Damage Caused by Obesity. (2017, June 28). CardioSmart. https://www.cardiosmart.org/news/2017/6/exercise-minimizes-heart-damage-caused-by-obesity

Flegal, K. M., Kit, B. K., Orpana, H., & Graubard, B. I. (2013). *Association of All-Cause Mortality With Overweight and Obesity Using Standard Body Mass Index Categories*. JAMA, 309(1), 71. https://doi.org/10.1001/jama.2012.113905

Fogoros, R. N. (n.d.). *Why Being a Little Overweight May Be OK*. Verywell Health. https://www.verywellhealth.com/is-being-a-little-overweight-ok

Fuller, N. R., Burns, J., Sainsbury, A., Horsfield, S., da Luz, F., Zhang, S., Denyer, G., Markovic, T. P., & Caterson, I. D. (2017). *Examining the Association Between Depression and Obesity During a Weight Management Programme*. Clinical Obesity, 7(6), 354–359. https://doi.org/10.1111/cob.12208

Goldman, R. (2019, January 14). *Do You Have to Fast Before a Cholesterol Test?* Healthline. https://www.healthline.com/health/high-cholesterol/fast-before-cholesterol-test

Gunnars, K. (2014, March 30). *8 Common Diet and Wellness Myths*. Healthline. https://www.healthline.com/health-news/food-eight-wellness-myths-033014#8-Top-Wellness-Myths

Hegde, S. (2017, November 22). *Fasting Blood Sugar Test Procedure, Prep, Results Interpretation*. Health CheckUp.

https://www.healthcheckup.com/general/fasting-blood-sugar-test

Hendrick, B. (2011, February). *Obesity Increases Risk of Deadly Heart Attacks.* WebMD. https://www.webmd.com/heart-disease/news/20110214/obesity-increases-risk-of-deadly-heart-attacks

Holm, G. (2016). *T3 Test: Purpose, Procedure, & Risks.* Healthline. https://www.healthline.com/health/t3

How Does Obesity Cause Cancer? (2018, September 6). Cancer Research UK. https://www.cancerresearchuk.org/health-professional/awareness-and-prevention/obesity-and-cancer-information-for-health-professionals/how-does-obesity-cause-cancer

How Does Obesity Cause Type-2 Diabetes. (2018, July 21). Vitagene. https://vitagene.com/blog/does-obesity-cause-type-2-diabetes/

How High Blood Pressure Can Affect the Body. (2022, January 14). Mayo Clinic. https://www.mayoclinic.org/diseases-conditions/high-blood-pressure/in-depth/high-blood-pressure/art-20045868

Intensive Behavioral Therapy for Obesity. (n.d.). John Hopkins Medicine. https://www.hopkinsmedicine.org/health/treatment-tests-and-therapies/intensive-behavioral-therapy-for-obesity

Kelly, C. (2021, January 20). *Obesity and Asthma—The Link, Risk Factors, and Management of Each.* Prescription Hope. https://prescriptionhope.com/blog-obesity-and-asthma

Khan, S. S., Ning, H., Wilkins, J. T., Allen, N., Carnethon, M., Berry, J. D., Sweis, R. N., & Lloyd-Jones, D. M. (2018). *Association of Body Mass Index With Lifetime Risk of Cardiovascular Disease and*

Compression of Morbidity. JAMA Cardiology, 3(4), 280–287. https://doi.org/10.1001/jamacardio.2018.0022

Kucera, J. (2018, August 2). *Sleep Apnea and Obesity.* Obesity Medicine Association. https://obesitymedicine.org/sleep-apnea-and-obesity

Lewis, R. (2020). *Tom Arnold Loses a Full 100 Lbs.—and Isn't Afraid to Go Shirtless.* People Magazine. https://people.com/health/tom-arnold-loses-a-full-100-lbs-and-isnt-afraid-to-go-shirtless/

Lifestyle Changes for Heart Attack Prevention. (2015, July 31). American Heart Association. https://www.heart.org/en/health-topics/heart-attack/life-after-a-heart-attack/lifestyle-changes-for-heart-attack-prevention

Liposuction. (2019). Mayo Clinic. https://www.mayoclinic.org/tests-procedures/liposuction/about/pac-20384586

Liver Function Tests. (2015). Mayo Clinic. https://www.mayoclinic.org/tests-procedures/liver-function-tests/about/pac-20394595

Lorcaserin Uses, Side Effects, & Warnings. (n.d.). Drugs.com. https://www.drugs.com/mtm/lorcaserin.html

MacGill, M. (2022, March 9). *Gastric Bands: How It Works, Surgery, Who Should Have It.* Medical News Today. https://www.medicalnewstoday.com/articles/298313#risks

Marcin, A. (2018, August 6). *Does Hypnotherapy for Weight Loss Work?* Healthline. https://www.healthline.com/health/hypnotherapy-weight-loss#types

Mozo, M. V., Finucane, F. M., & Flaherty, G. T. (2017). *Health Challenges of International Travel for Obese Patients.* Journal of Travel Medicine, 24(6). https://doi.org/10.1093/jtm/tax065

Multum, C. (2020, December 17). *Liraglutide Uses, Side Effects, & Warnings.* Drugs.com. https://www.drugs.com/mtm/liraglutide.html

Newcomb, A., & Steinhilber, B. (2020, May 29). *Jessica Simpson Lost 100 Pounds—Three Times—With These Lifestyle Changes.* Today Magazine. https://www.today.com/health/jessica-simpson-weight-loss-trainer-harley-pasternak-reveals-how-she-t182690

Obesity and Overweight. (2021, June 9). World Health Organization. https://www.who.int/news-room/fact-sheets/detail/obesity-and-overweight

Obesity—Diagnosis and Treatment. (2021, September 2). Mayo Clinic. https://www.mayoclinic.org/diseases-conditions/obesity/diagnosis-treatment/drc-20375749

Obesity in Children and Teens. (2016, April). American Academy of Child and Adolescent Psychiatry. https://www.aacap.org/AACAP/Families_and_Youth/Facts_for_Families/FFF-Guide/Obesity-In-Children-And-Teens-079.aspx

Obesity, Race/Ethnicity, and COVID-19. (2020b, September 17). Centers for Disease Control and Prevention. https://www.cdc.gov/obesity/data/obesity-and-covid-19.html

Peeters A, Barendregt JJ, Willekens F, Mackenbach JP, Mamun AA, Bonneux L (2003) *Obesity in Adulthood and Its Consequences for Life Expectancy: A Life-Table Analysis.* Ann Intern Med.

Phelamei, S. (2020, September 28). *Heavy Meals Can Trigger a Heart Attack: Here's How to Prevent Overeating and Switch to a Heart-Healthy Diet.* Times Now News. https://www.timesnownews.com/health/article/heavy-meals-can-trigger-a-heart-attack-here-s-how-to-prevent-overeating-and-switch-to-a-heart-healthy-diet/659065

Pietrangelo, A. (2017). *Cholesterol and Heart Disease: Is There a Connection?* Healthline. https://www.healthline.com/health/cholesterol-and-heart-disease

Puhl, R., & Brownell, K. D. (2001). *Bias, Discrimination, and Obesity.* Obesity Research, 9(12), 788–805. https://doi.org/10.1038/oby.2001.108

Sengupta, S. (2018, March 14). *Obesity Diet: What To Eat and Avoid To Manage Obesity.* NDTV Food. https://food.ndtv.com/food-drinks/obesity-diet-what-to-eat-and-avoid-to-manage-obesity-1815463

Social Isolation, Obesity, and Health. (2013, August 29). ConscienHealth. https://conscienhealth.org/2013/08/social-isolation-obesity-health/

Staff, D. T. N. (2018, March 29). *Social Effects Of Type 2 Diabetes.* Diabetestalk.net. https://diabetestalk.net/diabetes/social-effects-of-type-2-diabetes

Stookey, J. D., Constant, F., Popkin, B. M., & Gardner, C. D. (2008). *Drinking Water Is Associated With Weight Loss in Overweight Dieting Women Independent of Diet and Activity.* Obesity, 16(11), 2481–2488. https://doi.org/10.1038/oby.2008.409

Stradling, J., Roberts, D., Wilson, A., & Lovelock, F. (1998). *Controlled Trial of Hypnotherapy for Weight Loss in Patients With Obstructive Sleep Apnea.* International Journal of Obesity and Related Metabolic

Disorders: Journal of the International Association for the Study of Obesity, 22(3), 278–281. https://doi.org/10.1038/sj.ijo.0800578

Suni, E. (2019). *Sleep Apnea.* National Sleep Foundation. https://www.sleepfoundation.org/sleep-apnea

Sutaria, S., Devakumar, D., Yasuda, S. S., Das, S., & Saxena, S. (2018). *Is Obesity Associated With Depression in Children?* Systematic Review and Meta-Analysis. Archives of Disease in Childhood, 104(1), archdischild-2017-314608. https://doi.org/10.1136/archdischild-2017-314608

10 Ways to Control High Blood Pressure Without Medication. (2019, January 9). Mayo Clinic. https://www.mayoclinic.org/diseases-conditions/high-blood-pressure/in-depth/high-blood-pressure/art-20046974

10 Weight-Loss Myths. (2021, November 25). NHS. https://www.nhs.uk/live-well/healthy-weight/managing-your-weight/ten-weight-loss-myths/

Thompson, J. (2021, December 27). *5 Pro Athletes Who Overcame Childhood Struggles With Diet and Fitness.* Insider Magazine. https://www.insider.com/pro-athletes-who-struggled-weight

Thornton, P. (2018). *Phentermine.* Drugs.com. https://www.drugs.com/phentermine.html

Three Ways Obesity Contributes to Heart Disease. (2019, March 25). Penn Medicine. https://www.pennmedicine.org/updates/blogs/metabolic-and-bariatric-surgery-blog/2019/march/obesity-and-heart-disease

Types of Bariatric Surgery. (2019, October 25). National Institute of Diabetes and Digestive and Kidney Diseases.

https://www.niddk.nih.gov/health-information/weight-management/bariatric-surgery/types

What is Obesity and Morbid Obesity? (n.d.). University Healthcare. https://www.universityhealth.org/wellness-tips-information/everyday-health/obesity-weight-management/about-morbid-obesity

World Obesity Atlas 2022. (2022). The World Obesity Federation. https://s3-eu-west-1.amazonaws.com/wof-files/World_Obesity_Atlas_2022.pdf

Yang, Y. C., McClintock, M. K., Kozloski, M., & Li, T. (2013). *Social Isolation and Adult Mortality.* Journal of Health and Social Behavior, 54(2), 183–203. https://doi.org/10.1177/0022146513485244

Image References

Alexandra Gorn. (2017, December 6). [*woman covering her face with blanket*] [Image]. Unsplash. https://unsplash.com/photos/smuS_jUZa9I

Andres Siimon. (2019, April 16). [*white cigarette stick on white wall*] [Image]. Unsplash. https://unsplash.com/photos/ryBnRg4c3L0

Bru-nO. (2019). [*Man measuring waist size*] [Image]. Pixabay. https://pixabay.com/photos/measuring-tape-measure-belly-thick-4590164/

Camila Quintero Franco. (2019, March 25). [*woman's portrait*] [Image]. Unsplash. https://unsplash.com/photos/mC852jACK1g

Edgar Chaparro. (2018, May 17). [*grayscale photo of man working out*] [Image]. Unsplash. https://unsplash.com/photos/sHfo3WOgGTU

Farhad Ibrahimzade. (2021, July 10). [*cooked food on white ceramic plate*] [Image]. Unsplash. https://unsplash.com/photos/0DOPpeJVVWQ

Freestocks. (2016, March 7). [*woman holding stomach—expecting*] [Image]. Unsplash. https://unsplash.com/photos/ux53SGpRAHU

i yunmai. (2018, April 4). [*person standing on white digital bathroom scales*] [Image]. Unsplash. https://unsplash.com/photos/5jctAMjz21A

James Yarema. (2020, May 6). [*white medication pills on brown surface*] [Image]. Unsplash. https://unsplash.com/photos/kdgiNc0sDeI

Marcel Heil. (2018, December 23). [*man eating hamburger*] [Image]. Unsplash. https://unsplash.com/photos/qbdiF4C28q4

Markus Winkler. (2020, June 8). [*black android smartphone on brown wooden table*] [Image]. Unsplash. https://unsplash.com/photos/bOhKb8e0Iks

Mockup Graphics. (2021, March 11). [*white and black digital device*] [Image]. Unsplash. https://unsplash.com/photos/i1iqQRLULlg

Mykenzie Johnson. (2020, June 30). [*black smartphone beside white plastic bottle and black sugar tester*] [Image]. Unsplash. https://unsplash.com/photos/4qjxCUOc3iQ

Myriam Zilles. (2020, December 10). [*white blue and orange medication pills*] [Image]. Unsplash. https://unsplash.com/photos/KltoLK6Mk-g

Nguyễn Hiệp. (2021, March 11). [*person in white long sleeve shirt sitting on chair*] [Image]. Unsplash. https://unsplash.com/photos/2rNHliX6XHk

Piron Guillaume. (2017, December 28). [*gray surgical scissors near doctor in operating room*] [Image]. Unsplash. https://unsplash.com/photos/iwzaTMpBD7Q

Shelley Pauls. (2020, June 8). [*green and red vegetable on brown wooden table*] [Image]. Unsplash. https://unsplash.com/photos/Zaiuy5dKeCk

Sincerely Media. (2022, February 19). [*breathing equipment for asthma*] [Image]. Unsplash. https://unsplash.com/photos/Vs6FihuzxCg

Sydney Sims. (2018, January 18). [*person holding white printer paper*] [Image]. Unsplash. https://unsplash.com/photos/fZ2hMpHIrbI

Towfiqu Barbhuiya. (2021, October 17). [*person squeezing stomach roll*] [Image]. Unsplash. https://unsplash.com/photos/J6g_szOtMF4